The Garden Apothecary

Transform Flowers, Weeds and Plants into Healing Remedies

BECKY COLE

Hardie Grant

BOOKS

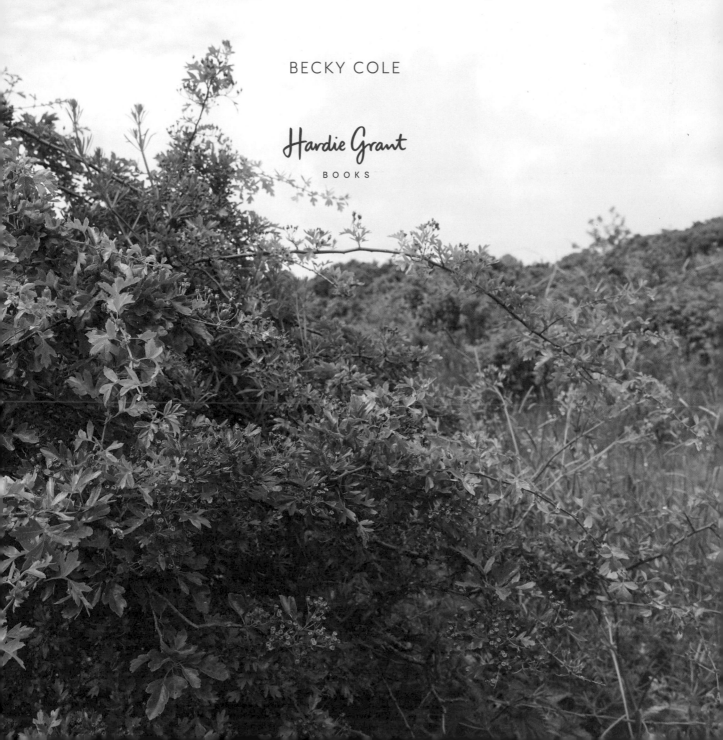

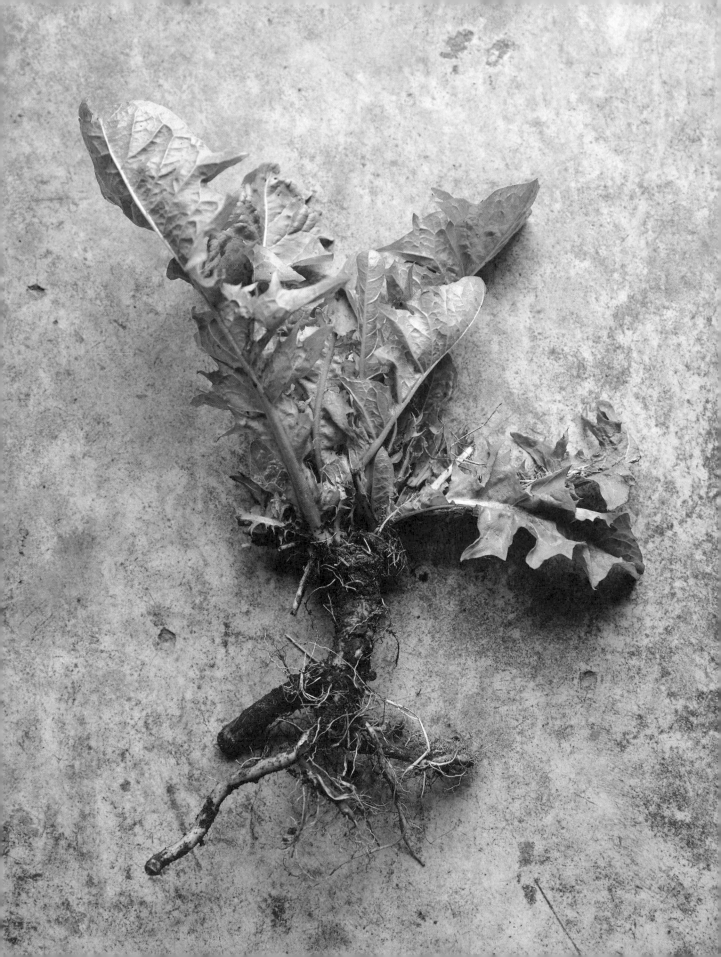

Contents

The Wild Garden

In my early years as a novice gardener, I would wrestle with garden weeds, waging what seemed like an impossible war against nature itself. Stubbornly hacking away at them with my blunt trowel and assailing them with choice expletives, I'd promise myself that I would finally get on top of it all and my garden would one day be weed-free. However, my enthusiasm soon waned and using a toxic weedkiller was never an option for me, so I finally stopped battling. I let go of the fantasy of a perfect carpet of velvety lawn and I downed tools. I put everything on pause and began to look around my garden as if for the first time. Surely a native hedgerow dotted with red hawthorn berries and tangled with honeysuckle would be easier and more beautiful than sweating over the prescribed clipped privet hedge? Or maybe that patch of determined nettles could actually be beneficial not only to the soil and local wildlife but also to my health?

Deciding to learn more, I began the first of many years of herbal study. I discovered with utter childlike joy that many of the weeds that kept popping up in my garden actually had incredible and much needed medicinal uses. That bed of nettles was actually rich in minerals and an amazing tonic for restoring general health to the body as well as enriching the soil. Dandelion was an under-utilised spring green, delicious sautéed for lunch and also beneficial as a liver tonic. Plantain became the herb I reached out for to soothe pesky splinters and other sore skin complaints. I started to notice the self-heal (*Prunella vulgaris*) plant that grew around the periphery of my lawn and almost cried with joy when a rogue clump of oats (*Avena sativa*) began to grow in a neglected, overgrown flowerbed. The chickweed (*Stelleria media*) that enjoyed sprawling over my vegetable beds in the polytunnel was now no longer thrown onto the compost heap but rather gathered into my garden trug and brought home to be blitzed into a delicious pesto or soaked in oil to make the perfect baby balm for my newborn.

My wild hedgerow not only protects me from the salty winds that batter the Atlantic coast here in County Antrim, Ireland, but also supplies me with a rich source of herbal medicines. It has been shown that the abundant, antioxidant-rich berries of the hawthorn and elder can indeed gently boost our health during those challenging winter months. The spring greens such as dandelion (*Urtica dioica*), cleavers (*Galium aparine*) and chickweed that grow in the shelter of the hedge provide a gentle detox to the body and a tonic when used in infused vinegars and teas. In summer, the abundance of blossom calls for heart medicine – flower essences to shift energy, blossoms tinctured and edible flowers made into the ultimate celebratory food.

Inspired by this new approach I also changed my doorstep container garden, filling the tubs with fragrant herbs and edible flowers such as pelargoniums, daisies, violas and calendula. This looks just as pretty as before, only now I can grab a bunch of rosemary or sage without having to find my wellies first. Each cake I bake for our farm shop now wears a crown of bright petals, bringing joy to all the senses!

Working with nature and the seasons, rather than trying to control and exploit my garden, has led me to a new respect for all those once problematic weeds. Living sustainably and in tune with nature is at the very heart of well-being. I hope this book will inspire you to see your garden and the plants around you with fresh eyes.

Here's to embracing the weeds!

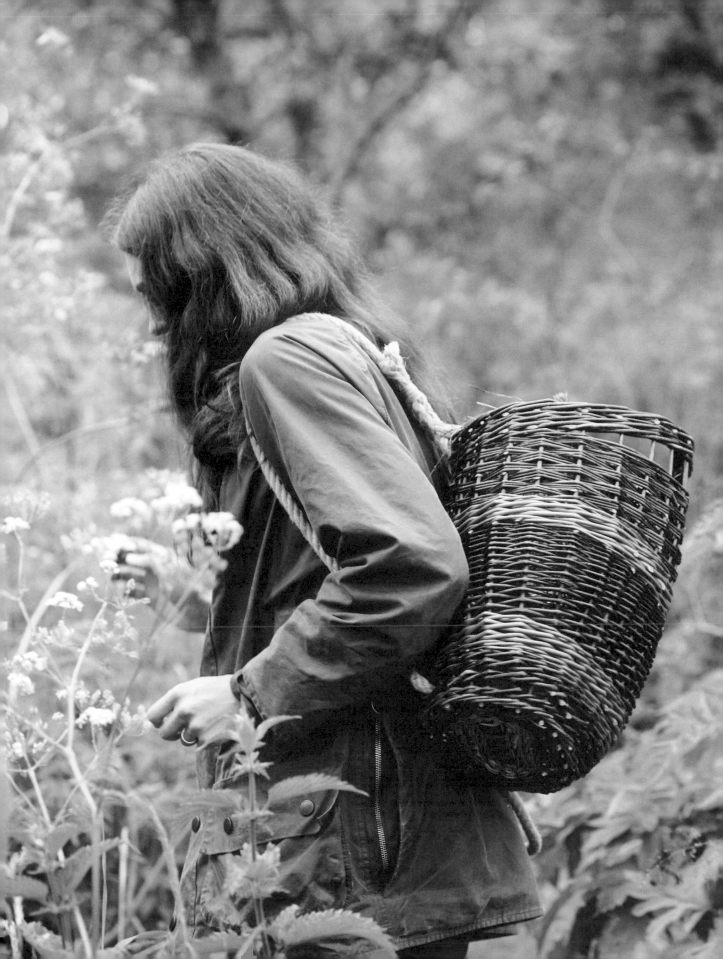

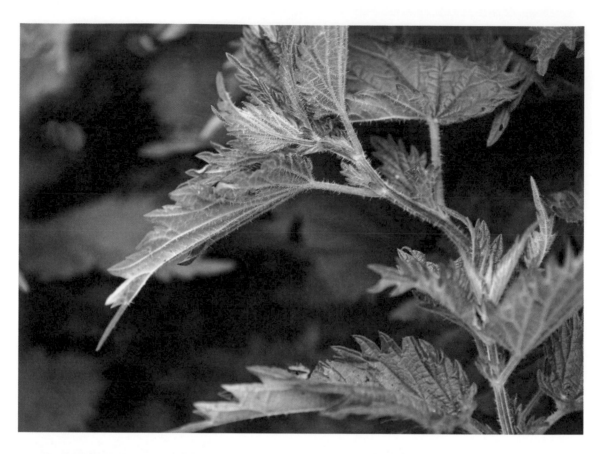

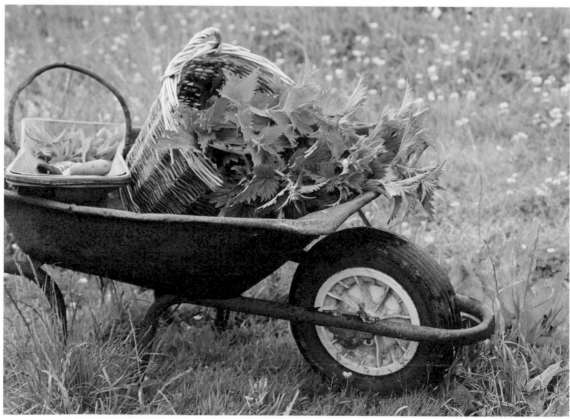

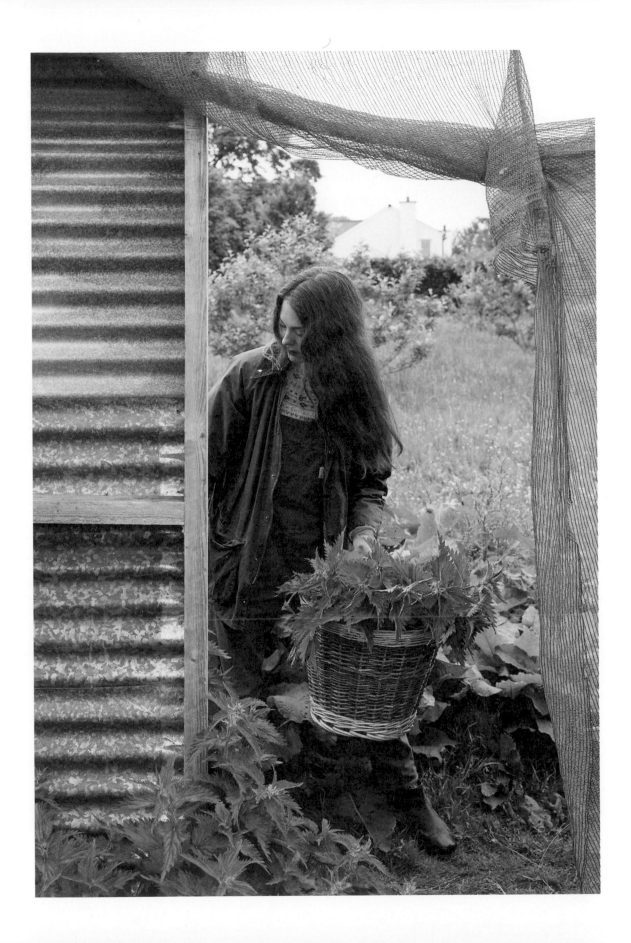

How to Use This Book

Welcome to *The Garden Apothecary*! I am really looking forward to sharing the techniques of a herbalist with you and showing you the alchemy that can come straight from your very own garden.

This book is mainly divided into techniques and plant profiles. In the techniques chapter, I share how to create the master recipes you will need in order to make the recipes that are dotted throughout the plant profiles. I suggest you start with the section on Infusions & Decoctions (see pages 31–35). This contains the basic method for making a water-based infusion (otherwise known as a tea), which is actually the backbone of creating almost every herbal remedy. Once you've mastered this skill, you'll find the others, such as making a syrup, a cinch. If you'd rather jump straight into the herbal profiles, then you can always revisit the techniques chapter later when you fancy making a remedy. I suggest you check your chosen recipe first in case you need to make a herbal infusion or oil in advance, as this process can take a number of weeks.

There are 20 plant profiles in this book. I've selected some of the most common and safest herbs that I know and ones I really love working with. You'll recognise most of them as garden weeds, but I hope you'll be excited to learn their incredible medicinal properties and uses and come to enjoy them as much as I do!

Each herb is listed according to its Latin name, which is really important as some plants have similar common names. Always work with the Latin name when using plants for medicine. The inclusion of the plant family will also help with identification and build your foraging skills. The 'Parts used' lets you know which parts of the plant are used for herbal medicine – for some plants it will just be their leaves, while for others it may be the root. Not all parts of the plant will be usable. For example, while I use the flowers and berries of the elder tree, it would not be advisable for new herbalists to use the leaves, roots and bark as these can be highly toxic.

In the plant profiles I've also included the 'energetics' of each plant, which can be helpful when selecting herbs for specific conditions. The energetics of the herbs is a subtle way of pairing the correct herb with a person. For example, you may have a cough and want a herb to help support your healing. While there are plenty of herbs that could be used for this, if you dig a little deeper you will find that the cough could be categorised as hot or cold and also dry or damp. If your cough is hot and damp, you want a herb that will not only target the respiratory system but also has cooling and drying qualities. In contrast, if the cough is cold and dry, the herb(s) you need will be warming and moistening.

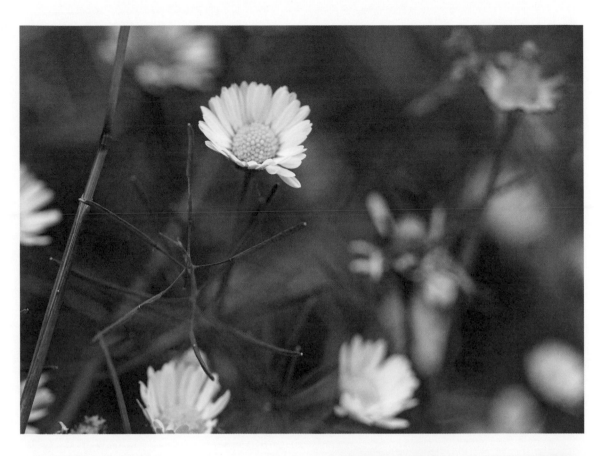

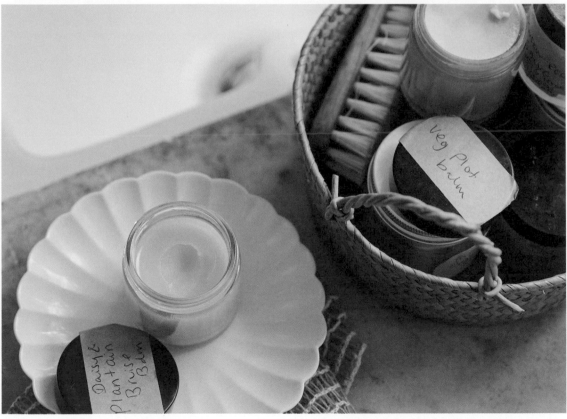

The 'actions' of each herb is where you will find what each can be used for. It may have antimicrobial qualities, perhaps be carminative or it could be a wonderful diaphoretic herb. Some of these terms might be new to you, in which case you will find a more in-depth description of each action in the Glossary on page 171. Most herbs have multiple actions, which means they have many uses.

Every herb has its own introduction where I share my favourite uses for each as well as its medicinal effects. I have also included some basic identification notes but, as this is not a foraging guide, I strongly suggest you pick up a botanical identification book with fine detail so you can cross-reference and make sure you are picking the right thing. I have shared some of my favourite foraging guides in the Resources section at the back of the book.

There are also some notes on how and when to harvest particular herbs correctly. This is vital to ensure you pick the herbs when they are at their most potent. Most herbs are at their best between spring and autumn, although pine and some of the kitchen herbs, such as thyme, can also be found during winter.

Finally, after each plant profile there are a handful of recipes to try out. Almost all of these can be adapted to suit you and what is available to you. Feel free to omit or swap out certain herbs. As long as you use the energetics and actions as a reference you can't go too wrong! I like to keep notes in my *Materia medica* (see page 21) as I blend and make up herbal medicine, and I recommend you do the same. This way you can easily remember what substitute worked well and keep records of favourite recipes and herbs.

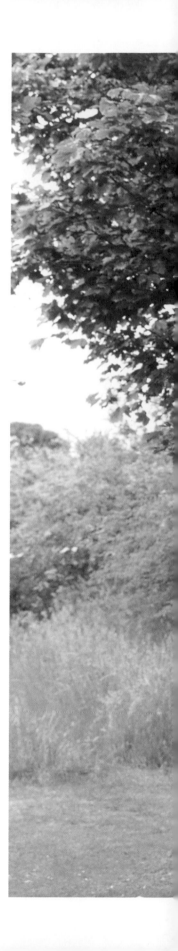

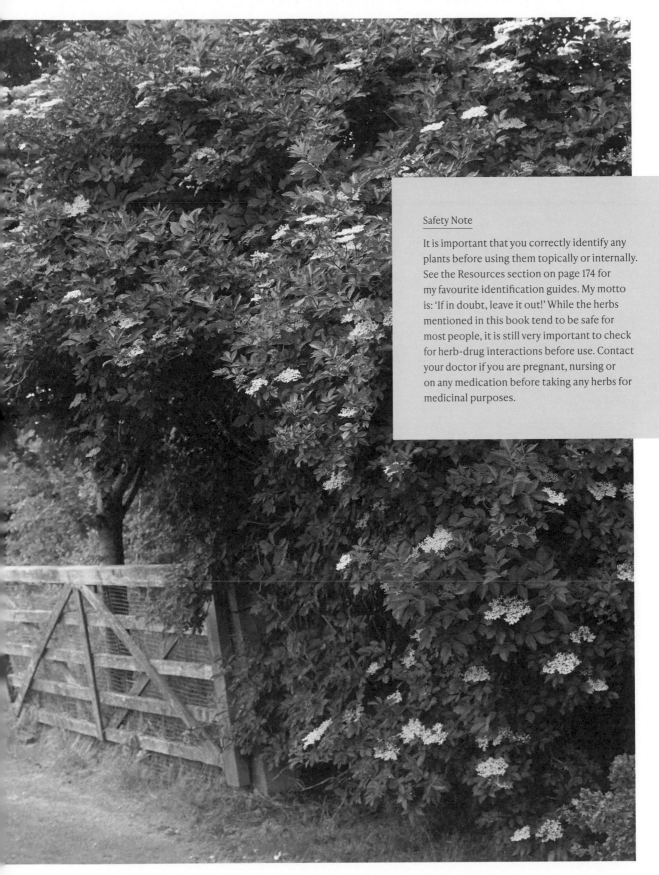

Safety Note

It is important that you correctly identify any plants before using them topically or internally. See the Resources section on page 174 for my favourite identification guides. My motto is: 'If in doubt, leave it out!' While the herbs mentioned in this book tend to be safe for most people, it is still very important to check for herb-drug interactions before use. Contact your doctor if you are pregnant, nursing or on any medication before taking any herbs for medicinal purposes.

Chapter One

Herbs & Herbalism

Have you ever taken elderberry syrup
or sipped on a cold elderflower cordial?
Maybe you've used spices such as
cinnamon and turmeric in your cooking?
If that's the case, you have already been
using herbs and enjoying their benefits.

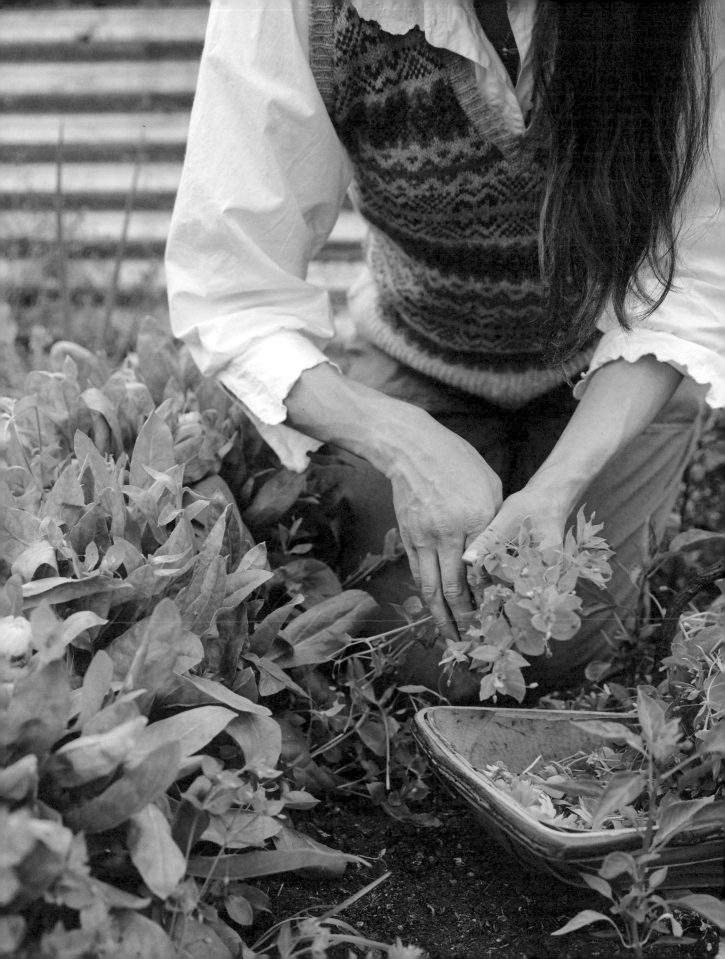

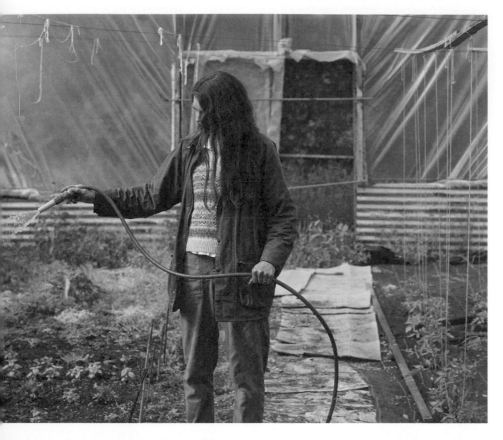
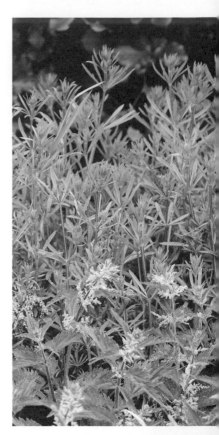
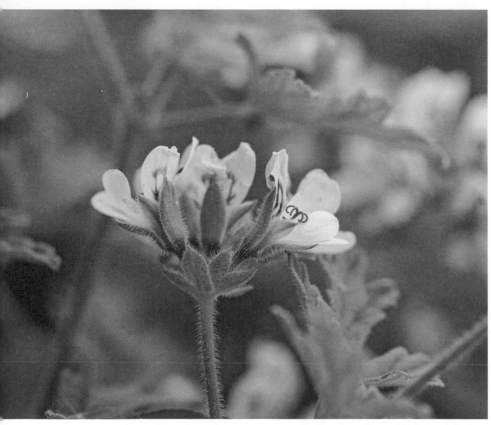
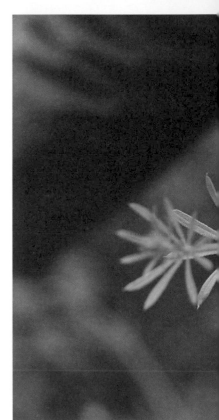

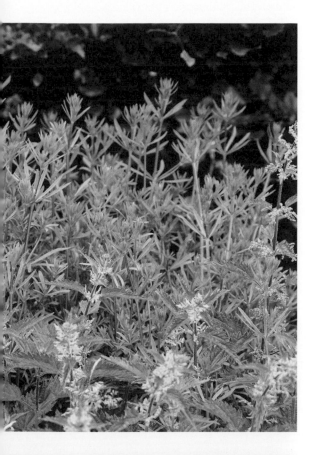

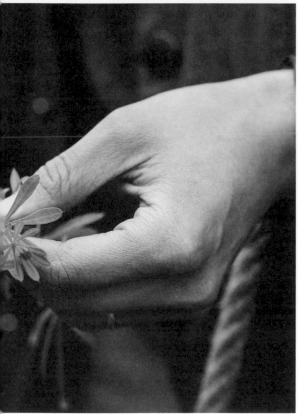

When we think of herbs, we tend to focus on culinary herbs such as rosemary, thyme and sage which are commonly used in cooking.

However, most herbalists also place any plant with useful medicinal qualities in that category. To me, herbs are plants that promote wellness in some way, such as easing the symptoms of colds and sniffles. Or to boost my immunity or mood during mid-winter. Each herb has its own individual properties which can be harnessed through the alchemic-like creation of herbal remedies.

If you are a gardener, you already know the joy that comes from tending your garden through the year. Working in the garden, whether burying your hands in compost to plant seeds in spring or pruning in autumn, builds a connection not only with the plants themselves, but also with the soil, local wildlife and the seasons. This relationship can be further enriched through learning about the uses of herbs and how to turn your garden into your very own wild apothecary. By growing herbs that you will later harvest, dry and use for syrups, teas and tinctures, you will open up a whole new dimension in the world of plants and gardening.

Herbalism is a skill that we can all learn and benefit from. By growing and harvesting our own medicinal plants we can support our health naturally while saving some money at the same time. Herbalism encourages us to learn about how our body works and how best to maintain our health. Herbalism can bring powerful knowledge and skills to our homes as well as help us to create a more self-sufficient garden.

GROWING HERBS

The thought of growing my own herbs captivated my imagination many years ago. The dream of enjoying a cup of home-grown lemon balm tea on a summer's evening was one of my goals when we moved into our farm cottage. Since that initial thought, I've grown many herbs from seed and finally built up a decent collection of mint plants. My herb garden is a little scattered – there's fennel growing in my back garden, chamomile by my doorstep and calendula down by the polytunnels. However, what I've learnt through the process is that it's possible to grow herbs in most places, from a garden bed to a windowsill. Whatever space you have, you can enjoy a cup of home-grown herbal tea.

If you have a small outdoor space or balcony, then containers such as terracotta pots are your best bet for an abundant herb garden. In all honesty, I find that I opt for my doorstep herbs far more than the ones I grow in my main garden as they are within arm's reach. Most of the herbs mentioned in this book will flourish in a container. Just make sure your chosen container has drainage holes and provides enough space for the plant.

Wild herbs like nettle, cleavers, plantain and chickweed can also be grown from seed, although you might find them appearing in parts of your garden without any invitation!

Hawthorn, pine and elder are bigger plants and can grow into large trees if left unchecked, but if you have a big enough container and the space, there is no reason why you can't grow these – even on a modest balcony.

For those without this amount of outdoor space, then a window box inside or outside is a good option. I often plant nasturtium, calendula and chamomile, as well as kitchen herbs like rosemary, thyme and mint, in window boxes and, while they will never become large plants, they will happily grow and provide you with a decent harvest of leaves or flowers. Lavender also looks beautiful in a window box and some dwarf varieties work well as houseplants, too.

If you want to go all out and grow a garden bed full of herbs, then the world is your oyster. Consider essential factors like soil type and light levels and then choose herbs that will flourish in your location. Be careful when planting mint directly in the bed, however, as it does love to take over large patches of garden, so should be contained in a pot.

Edible Flowers

Although the main focus of this book is herbal remedies, I had to give a mention to edible flowers. There is something so visually pleasing about using edible flowers, they are a sort of soul medicine as such. Of course, some of the flowers will also have medicinal properties, such as nasturtium flowers (see page 156), but in general their beauty and energetics are their main benefits. There are so many edible flowers to try but some reliable ones include cornflower (*Centaurea cyanus*), borage (*Borago officinalis*), scented geraniums (*Pelargonium* spp.), lilac (*Syringa vulgaris*) and violet (*Viola* spp.) to name just a few. There are so many ways in which you can use edible flowers, including as a decoration, crystallised, in flower sugars, infused into honey, as syrups, oils, cordials, hot and cold infusions, in ice cubes, salads, vinegars, in curd, sorbets, ice cream, wines and gin ... The list goes on!

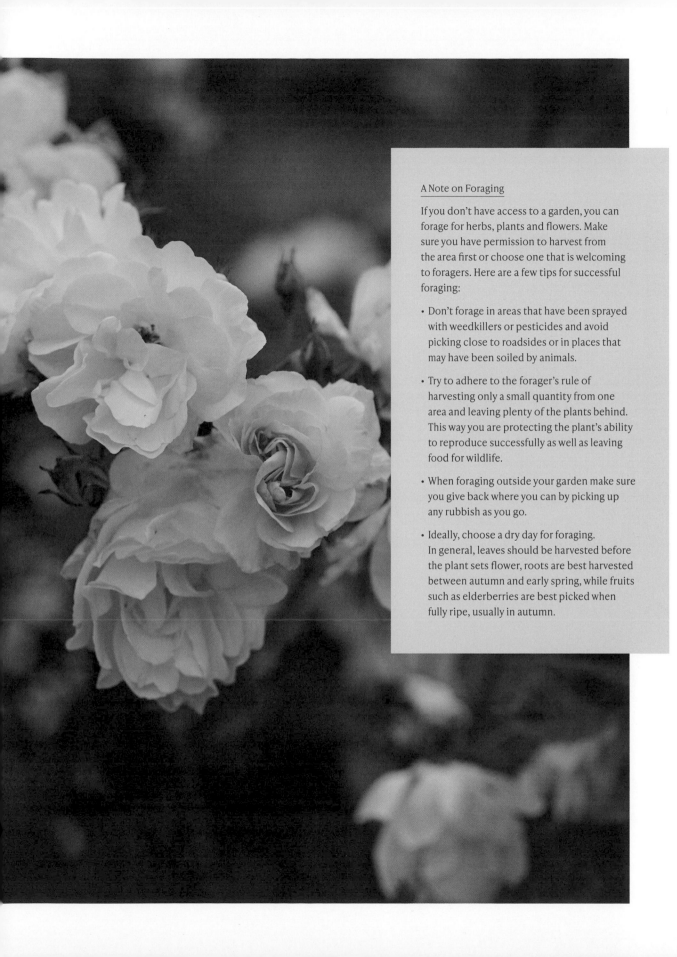

A Note on Foraging

If you don't have access to a garden, you can forage for herbs, plants and flowers. Make sure you have permission to harvest from the area first or choose one that is welcoming to foragers. Here are a few tips for successful foraging:

- Don't forage in areas that have been sprayed with weedkillers or pesticides and avoid picking close to roadsides or in places that may have been soiled by animals.

- Try to adhere to the forager's rule of harvesting only a small quantity from one area and leaving plenty of the plants behind. This way you are protecting the plant's ability to reproduce successfully as well as leaving food for wildlife.

- When foraging outside your garden make sure you give back where you can by picking up any rubbish as you go.

- Ideally, choose a dry day for foraging. In general, leaves should be harvested before the plant sets flower, roots are best harvested between autumn and early spring, while fruits such as elderberries are best picked when fully ripe, usually in autumn.

Chapter Two

The Home Apothecary

A home apothecary can be anything from a row of glass jars filled with dried herbs for teas to a cupboard of syrups, infusing tinctures, spiced vinegars and sweet herbal honeys.

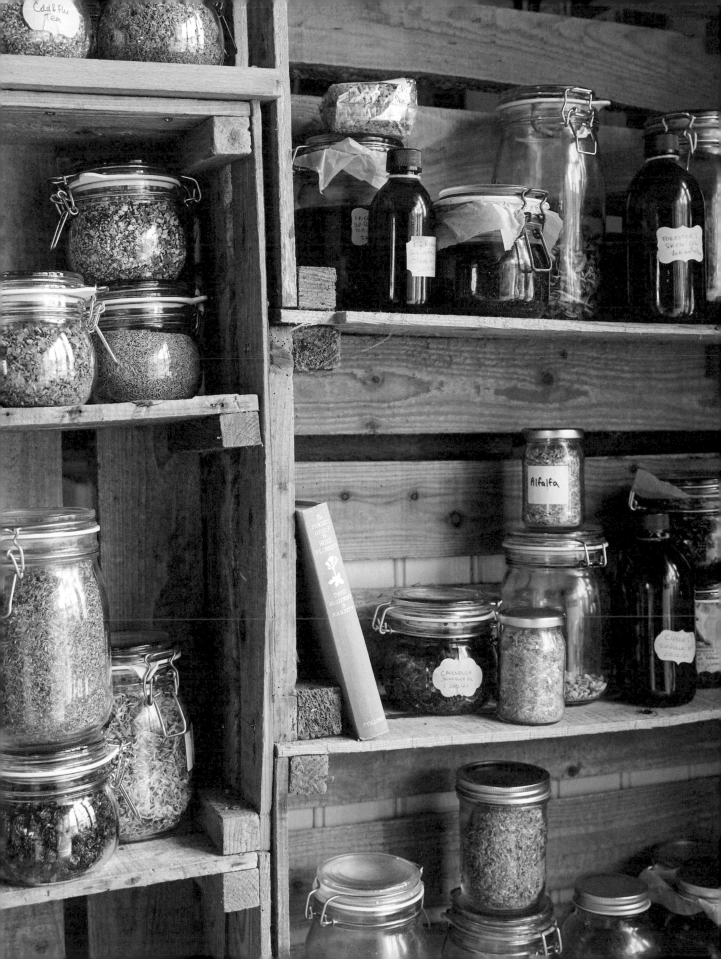

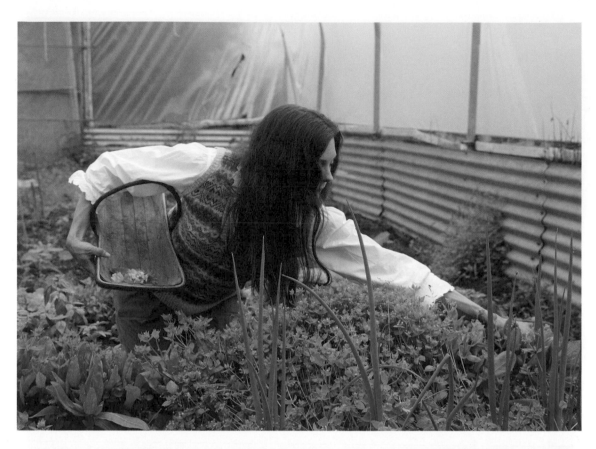

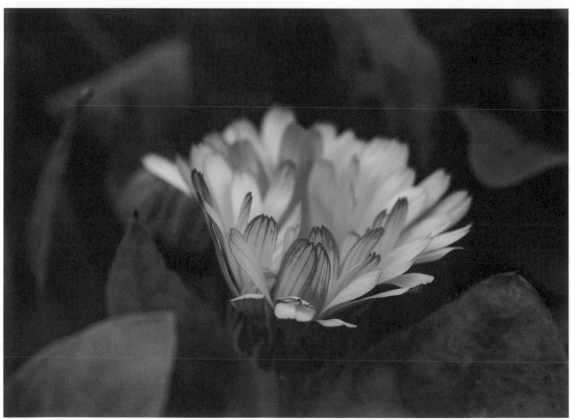

The exciting thing about creating a home apothecary is having the power to reach for a natural remedy when you need it. No trip to the shops required.

For example, if you find dozing off at night-time difficult, you can whip up a Chamomile Moon Milk (see page 69) to brew each evening. If you find yourself getting colds and sniffles often, then herbs such as rosemary, sage, thyme and nasturtium will feature prominently in your apothecary.

Knowing just a few key herbs and having the skills to make tried-and-tested recipes marks the start of a wonderful life as a home herbalist. Personally, I am never without jars of dried nettles, chamomile flowers, rose petals and elderberries. I often use fresh chickweed in my cooking and love those bitter spring greens when they're in season. I find my kitchen ebbs and flows with the seasons, and I adjust my remedies accordingly.

I like to take my time when learning about a herb. I start by making a study of its botanical details such as leaf shape, flowers and growing habit, ensuring that my identification is correct. Then I move on to its taste and scent by brewing a cup of tea with the herb and learning how it works medicinally. This is a perfect way to get to know a herb thoroughly. It is a good idea to create your own *Materia medica*, which is a sort of herbal journal containing your own sketches, notes and recipes.

I suggest that you read through the plant profiles and find a few that really resonate with you. Perhaps you've always been curious about a particular plant, or have certain ones growing in your garden already? Once you've chosen a few plants, you can move on to trying the different herbalist techniques as well as making some of the recipes I've shared. Remember to take notes on how you felt after using the recipes and how the herb is working for you.

One of my favourite herbalist techniques for the beginner is a simple herbal tea. Quick and effective, this is the mainstay of my home apothecary and a delicious way of consuming herbs, whether fresh or dried. Once you've mastered herbal teas, you'll find syrups, vinegars, honeys and tinctures easy to conjure up at home, too.

EQUIPMENT & INGREDIENTS

You don't need to buy lots of special or expensive equipment
to make the wonderful remedies in this book. You'll probably have
most of the tools and other items in your kitchen already.

Equipment

DIGITAL SCALE: A must-have for measuring out various
ingredients.

DOUBLE BOILER/BAIN-MARIE: You can buy a double
boiler or make a DIY version (that is, a bain-marie).
You can either nest one saucepan inside another or rest a
heatproof bowl over the saucepan. The base saucepan will
contain simmering water. Ideal for making balms and salves.

FINE MUSLIN (CHEESECLOTH): Essential for
straining out oils, vinegars and tinctures.

FUNNEL: Ideal for pouring liquids into small bottles.

HEATPROOF GLASS MEASURING JUG: Helpful for
measuring as well as pouring remedies into jars and bottles.

JARS AND TINS: Useful for storing your remedies.
Always make sure these have an airtight lid.

LABELS: Essential to help you remember what's in
each bottle or jar and when the remedy was made.

MEASURING CUPS AND SPOONS: Useful for measuring out
ingredients. I also recommend getting a small glass measuring
beaker for small quantities under 50 ml (1¾ fl oz/3 tablespoons).

MIXING BOWLS: A selection of glass or metal bowls is useful
when preparing ingredients.

NATURAL BAKING PARCHMENT: Useful for sealing lidded
jars when using vinegar or citrus juices, for example, which can
be corrosive.

PESTLE AND MORTAR: I like to use mine to mash up plants
for poultices and to grind up herbs and spices.

SEALABLE WIDE-MOUTHED JARS: Large jars such
as Kilner and Mason jars are ideal for storing remedies while
they infuse. Make sure the jars have an airtight lid.

SILICONE MOULDS AND ICE-CUBE TRAYS:
These make useful containers when making bath melts.

TEA STRAINER: For making herbal teas.

Ingredients

ALCOHOL: A strong vodka is needed to create a tincture (ideally, at least 40% alcohol). Alcohol extracts the properties of the plant and preserves them. The tincture is then dosed out in small quantities and usually diluted in water before consuming.

BEESWAX: This is used to create balms and salves and also protects the skin by creating a barrier.

CANDELILLA WAX: This is an alternative to beeswax for those who are avoiding animal products. It is harder than beeswax, so you'll want to use less of it in your products.

CARRIER OILS: These are oils derived from the seeds or flesh of a plant. They have properties that are beneficial to skin. Examples include olive oil, sunflower oil and jojoba oil. Make sure you source organic and unrefined oils. I use these to create infused oils.

ESSENTIAL OILS: Essential oils are very concentrated and aromatic plant extracts. They need diluting before use but can amp up the plant power of topical products.

GLYCERIN: Vegetable glycerin can be used as an alternative to vodka in tincture-making to create a glycerite. Make sure you're using a glycerin that is safe for ingestion. Glycerites are better suited to children and those sensitive to the alcohol used in tinctures.

HERBS: These are the star ingredients of the apothecary. I like to work mainly with dried herbs as these have a longer shelf life.

HONEY: Honey is used to make herbal-infused honeys, which are such a treat. I recommend using a local raw honey, which contains all its wonderful health benefits.

HYDROSOL: A hydrosol is plant-infused water which is the by-product of the essential oil distillation process. These waters contain some of the therapeutic properties of essential oils, but on a much milder scale.

PLANT BUTTERS: These are nourishing and softening for the skin and are naturally derived from the fatty parts of plants. They also contain specific vitamins and have different properties. Examples include shea butter and cocoa butter. I use them in balms.

VINEGAR: An organic raw apple cider vinegar that still contains the 'mother' is an essential for the home herbalist. This is used to create herbal-infused vinegars, which are very healthy for the system and can be used both internally and topically.

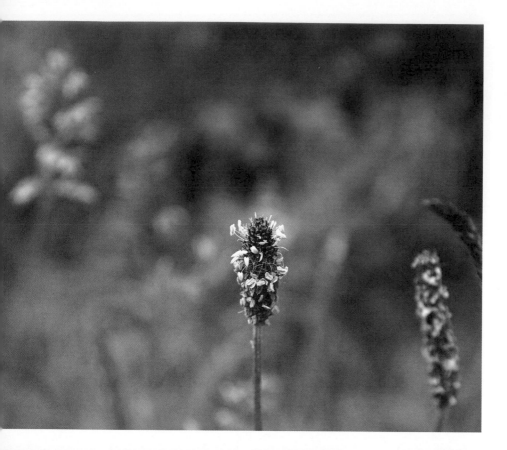

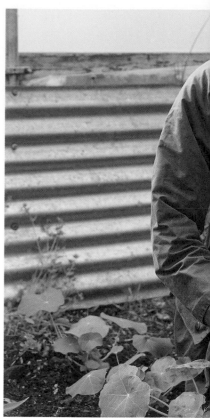

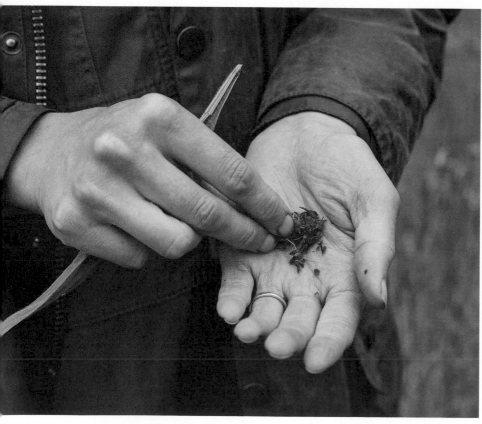

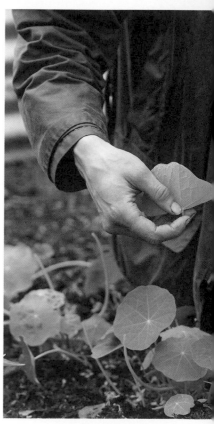

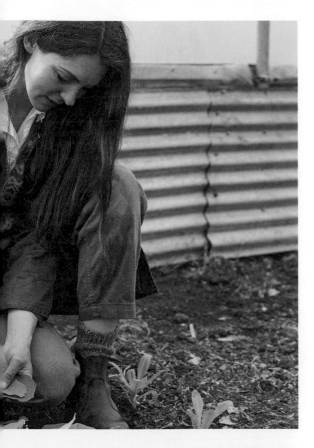

HARVESTING & DRYING

Part of the joy of making your own remedies is spending time outdoors harvesting the herbs. Once harvested, the herbs need to be sorted and dried (although you can also use them fresh in some recipes).

Harvesting Herbs

Herbs should be harvested on a dry day, when there is no water remaining on the plant. Ideally, harvest on a bright morning after the dew has lifted, but if this doesn't suit, just harvest whenever the opportunity arises.

In general, you should harvest the aerial (above-ground) parts of a herb before it flowers. Check the plant over, making sure of its identity and looking at how healthy it is. You'll want to ensure the leaves are fresh and disease free. Cut long stems of the herb near a node. This works particularly well for strong-stemmed plants such as rosemary and lemon balm which dry well in bundles. For herbs from which you just want the leaves, gently remove as many as you need, making sure you don't overharvest. An over-harvested plant will struggle.

Roots will need to be dug up carefully and are best harvested during autumn and spring, when they contain the most nutrients. I tend to leave roots alone during the summer months, when most of the plant's energy is going into the production of flowers, and during the winter when it's harder to identify plants due to the dieback of leaves.

I like to use a wide wicker basket when harvesting as this allows the plants to remain in good condition and prevents bruising, which often happens if you harvest into small bags.

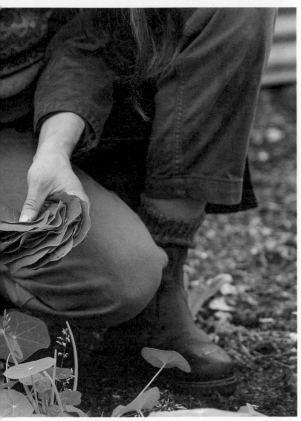

Sorting & Cleaning

Once you've harvested the herbs it's time to get garbling! Garbling is the process of sorting through the herbs, removing unwanted or damaged parts, soil or debris and any insects. As I harvest from my own land, I rarely wash leaves, flowers or aerial parts as this adds moisture and can also weaken some of the aromatic parts, especially the flowers. I should stress that it is essential you harvest plants that haven't been sprayed or been in contact with pesticides. If necessary, leaves can be washed carefully before use. Roots will need a very good wash and scrub, as they will be caked in mud. A small bristle brush is the best tool to ensure that all the soil is removed.

Preparation & Drying

Once your herbs are clean and sorted it is time to prepare them for drying. I like to dry herbs from my garden, as once dried the herbs can be stored for at least a year in an airtight jar, meaning I can work with a summer herb even in the midst of winter. One of the prettiest and most popular ways to dry herbs is the bundle method. This works well for herbs with long, strong stems and in homes that aren't damp. If you have a wood-burning stove, you can hang these bundles close by to benefit from the dry climate created by the fire.

To bundle, grab about five stems and secure them with an elastic band. Hang the bundles from a long piece of twine. (Using more than five stems may lead to the inner part of the bundle retaining moisture.)

I like to dry flower heads and smaller plant parts in a tray or wide basket. Lay out the clean herbs in one layer (any deeper and mould could grow) and place the tray or basket somewhere dry and warm until the herbs are dry. Try and avoid drying herbs in direct sunlight as this can affect their potency.

When preparing roots, chop them up into small, even slices or matchstick-like strips. These can be laid out on a tray or in a basket to dry but will take much longer than flowers and leaves to completely dry through.

If you live somewhere with a damp climate, you might find a food dehydrator a worthwhile purchase. This is a great way of quickly and successfully drying herbs and is my favourite method due to the wetter weather we have in Northern Ireland.

Herbs are ready to be stored as soon as they are completely dry, brittle and crumbly when rubbed between your palms. Roots will reduce in size, but it is important to cut one in half in order to check they are fully dried.

Crush any larger parts with your hands to reduce their size slightly and place in a clean, dry jar. Label the jar with the name of the herb and the date.

Leaves and aerial parts should last 1–2 years, whereas roots will last up to 2–3 years. You should discard herbs if they lose their colour or aromatic scent or become musty.

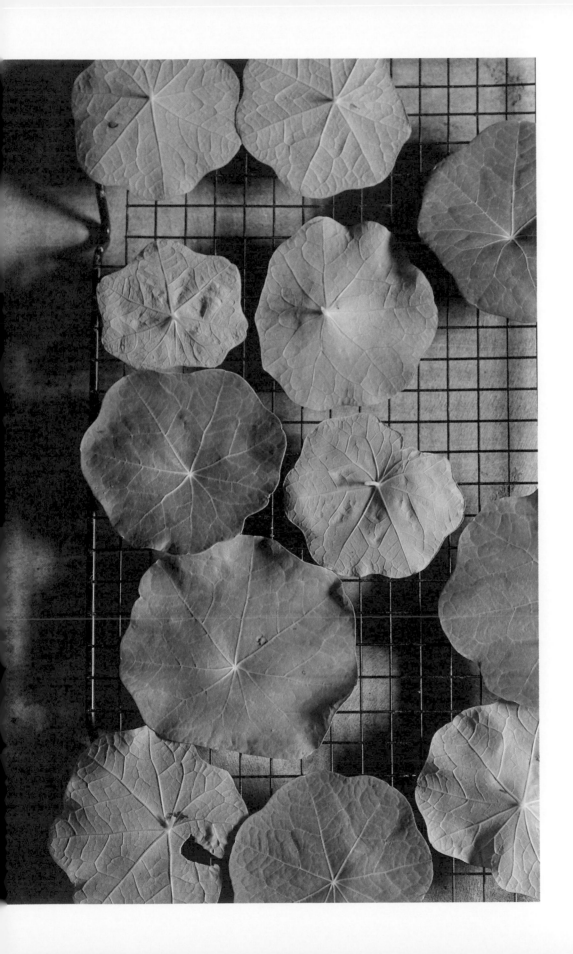

Chapter Three

Apothecary Techniques

Turning your home-grown herbs into plant-based remedies is much easier than you might think. While many herbalists gain a certain intuitive skill over time, we all begin in the same place, with a dose of curiosity and a love of plants.

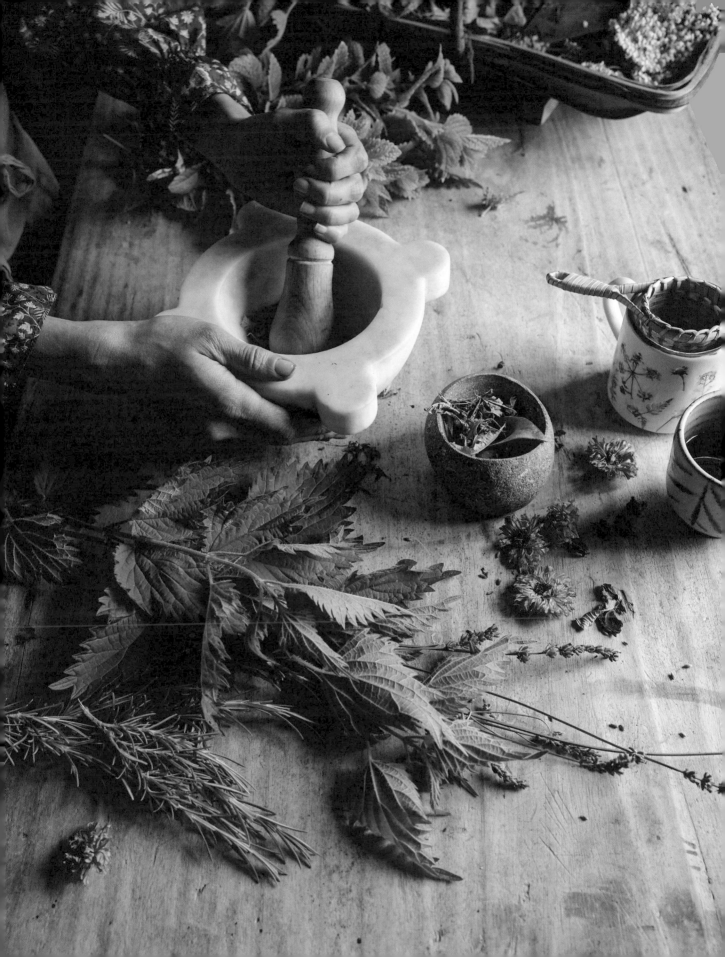

In this chapter, I will teach you how to create teas, vinegars, syrups, honeys, balms, tinctures and oils using traditional herbalist techniques. These beautiful medicines extract the beneficial properties and compounds of the plants and preserve them ready for consumption.

Different plants respond in different ways to the extraction method. For example, nettles work well in a vinegar extraction because the vinegar draws out and preserves their rich mineral content, while an alcohol-based tincture wouldn't be as effective. Marshmallow root is another herb that requires a specific extraction method. In this case, a water extraction (otherwise known as a tea) helps to make the most of all the wonderful mucilaginous properties of marshmallow root, while these roots wouldn't be as effective in a tincture. However, in general, the best approach is to be open to making mistakes and learning and taking notes as you go along.

Sterilising

It is important to sterilise storage jars and bottles before use, especially as many of your homemade remedies are made from organic ingredients and will be kept for up to a year. The best way to sterilise jars and bottles is to wash them in very hot, soapy water and then dry them in the oven at a low temperature.

INFUSIONS & DECOCTIONS

My favourite place to start when discovering new herbs and their medicinal properties is through a beautiful cup of herbal tea, otherwise known as a herbal infusion. A herbal infusion is simply herbs brewed in water for a set amount of time. The herbs are then strained from the liquid and the herbal water is enjoyed. This water contains herbal properties from the plant, giving our bodies a natural boost.

The infusion method is a quick and effective way of tasting and learning about a herb. You'll get a sense of the whole herb, from its flavour and scent to its benefits, and you'll be getting some extra hydration, too!

A herbal infusion is a relatively quick brew and works particularly well to soothe the mind and spirit as well as for medicinal needs. In general, a herbal infusion uses 1–2 teaspoons of dried herbs added to a mug of boiling water (around 250 ml/8½ fl oz/1 cup) and is infused for approximately 10 minutes. It's suitable for leaves, flowers and aromatic herbs and one I turn to daily for a boost in the morning or to calm down ready for bed at night. A herbal infusion is also the best option for chamomile, which can become bitter if overbrewed in a medicinal infusion (which has a longer infusion time) or a decoction (see right).

In general, I like to brew a big batch of herbal infusion and store the extra in the fridge to drink throughout the day to shift the symptoms I'm dealing with. Simply increase the quantities of herbs and water using the same ratio as for a standard infusion if you want to make more than one mug. Once brewed the infusion will last between 1–2 days in the fridge.

You can amp up the power of the herbal infusion by adding extra herbs (1 tablespoon per mug) and allowing a longer infusion time, approximately 20–30 minutes. This stronger infusion, often called a medicinal infusion, is one to reach for when you have a specific issue you need support with, such as a head cold.

An overnight infusion is my favourite way of utilising the properties of tonic herbs like nettle. Add 2–3 heaped tablespoons to 1 litre (34 fl oz/4 cups) of hot or cold water and infuse for at least eight hours or overnight. An overnight infusion is suitable for tonic herbs like nettle and oat straw and the long brewing time helps to extract every bit of the plant's medicine, making it a brilliant morning drink or addition to a smoothie.

A solar infusion (or sun tea) uses the power of the sun to gently infuse the herbs into the water. Add a teaspoon or tablespoon of herbs to a mug of cool water and allow it to be heated by the sun for 4–8 hours. A solar infusion is suitable for leaves, flowers such as lavender and rose, and aromatic herbs. This tea is a beautiful way to celebrate the summer season. There's nothing quite like sipping a gently warmed solar infusion to appreciate the beauty of the garden and the magic of mid-summer.

A decoction is the best way to extract the herbal goodness from the tougher parts of plants, such as roots, seeds, bark and dried fruits. For a decoction, you add a teaspoon or tablespoon of the plant material (depending on the strength you want) to 250 ml/8½ fl oz/1 cup of water and simmer in a saucepan for 20 minutes. Remove from the heat and leave to infuse for a further 20 minutes.

Note: If using fresh herbs for any of the above infusions, you might want to double the quantity. Dried herbs are more concentrated, so you will need more of the fresher material to get a similar effect.

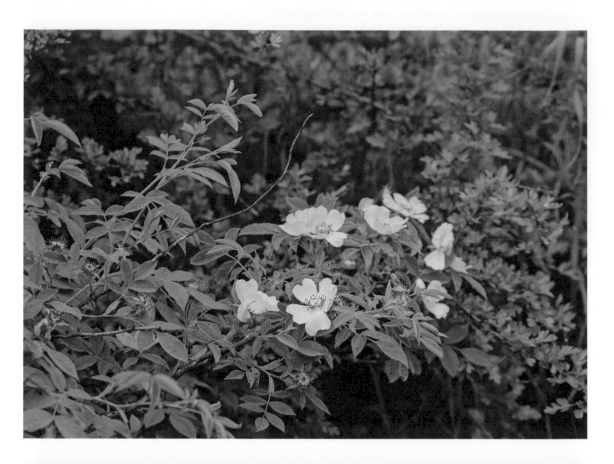

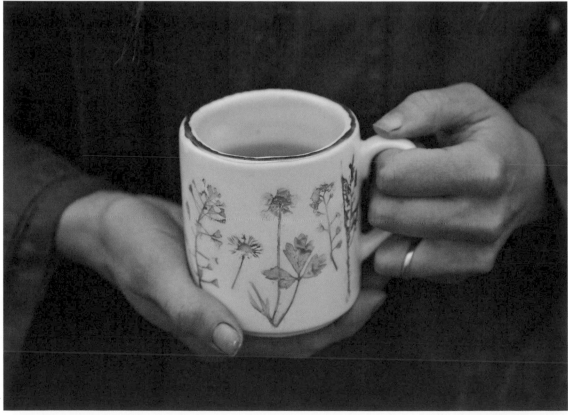

Infusion & Decoction Chart

Infusion/Decoction	Quantity	Water	Infusing time
Herbal infusion	1–2 teaspoons	250 ml/8½ fl oz/ 1 cup	10 minutes
Medicinal infusion	1 tablespoon	250 ml/8½ fl oz/ 1 cup	20–30 minutes
Overnight infusion	2–3 heaped tablespoons	1 litre/34 fl oz/ 4 cups	8 hours or overnight
Solar infusion	1 teaspoon or 1 tablespoon	250 ml/8½ fl oz/ 1 cup	4–8 hours in the sun
Decoction	1 teaspoon or 1 tablespoon	250 ml/8½ fl oz/ 1 cup	40 minutes (20 minutes simmering, 20 minutes infusing)

Infusions & Decoctions in this Book

How to Make a Herbal Infusion

YOU WILL NEED

Your choice of herbs
Boiling water
Honey or sweetener of choice (optional)
Tea strainer
Mug

METHOD

1. Place the dried or fresh herb in a mug (you can use a teapot or heatproof container if you want to make a larger amount). I often add the herb to a tea strainer and then place that inside my mug.

2. Pour over just-boiled water, covering all the herbs and filling the mug. Cover with a saucer to keep in the aromatics. If making a cold infusion, then simply pour over cold water instead of boiling water.

3. Allow to brew for the required time. Keep overnight brews in the fridge and solar infusions in direct sunlight. Strain out the herbs.

4. Stir in a teaspoon of honey (or similar), if needed, and enjoy.

How to Make a Herbal Decoction

YOU WILL NEED

Your choice of herbs
Water
Tea strainer or fine mesh sieve
Saucepan
Mug

METHOD

1. Put your herbs in a saucepan and pour over the required quantity of water. Place over the heat and bring to a simmer. Cover with a lid.

2. Simmer for 20 minutes, checking occasionally to make sure there is still water in the pan. If too much water has evaporated, just top up the pan with more.

3. Remove from the heat and, keeping the lid on, leave the decoction to infuse for a further 20 minutes.

4. Strain out the herbs and drink.

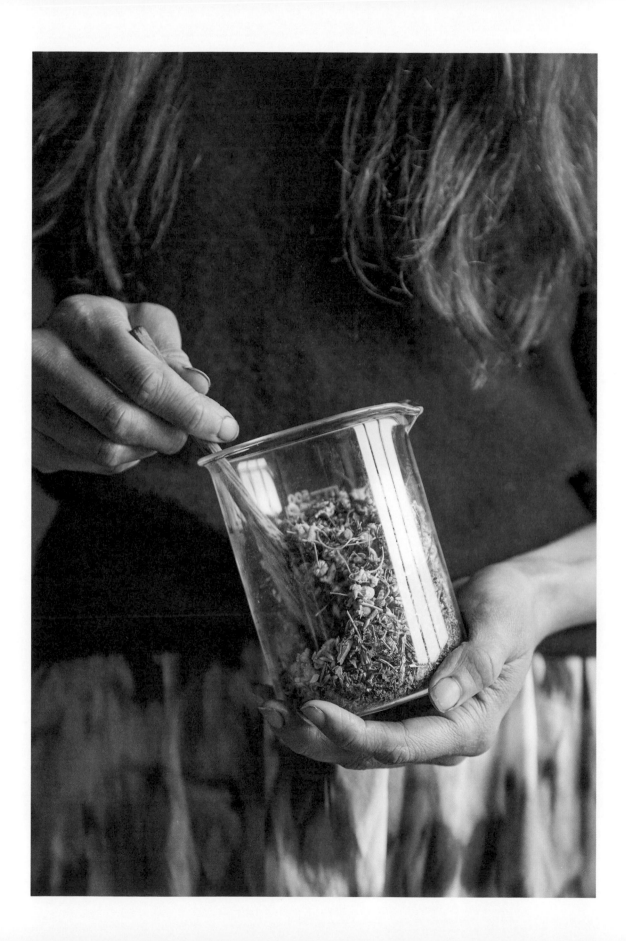

VINEGARS & OXYMELS

When I feel a cold coming on there is nothing quite like a cup of hot water with a big spoon of herbal vinegar or a sweetened oxymel stirred in. The hot steam and astringent vinegar work quickly at easing stuffed-up sinuses while the herbs work their magic.

Herbal-infused vinegars are a great way to create plant-based remedies that have a longer shelf life than infusions. Herbal vinegars are a combination of vinegar and herbs that are left to infuse over a few weeks. Just like the water used to make herbal infusions, the vinegar also extracts the plant constituents but, thanks to vinegar's shelf-stable qualities, a herbal vinegar will stay preserved for around a year if you are using dried herbs or up to three months with fresh.

Some plants are particularly well suited to a vinegar extraction, especially mineral-rich herbs like nettle. In fact, nettle is better extracted using vinegar than in an alcohol-based tincture. Other herbs that are well suited to vinegar are alkaloid-rich plants like oats.

Raw apple cider vinegar is my favourite vinegar to use due to its probiotic qualities. Look for a vinegar that includes the mother, as this will still contain all those beneficial properties. Vinegar is also known to be an antiseptic and supportive of digestion.

Vinegar can be a great alternative to alcohol-based tinctures for children or those avoiding alcohol. The herbal vinegar can be used as a tonic, diluted in warm water and sweetened if necessary. I'll often swap out a plain vinegar for a nettle vinegar for added benefits in a classic salad dressing. I also like to use herbal vinegars to clean the house, as a facial toner and as a hair and scalp tonic.

An oxymel is a honey-sweetened version of a herbal vinegar. It is made in a similar way to a herbal vinegar, but has the delicious addition of honey, too. It tastes tangy but also sweet and works well to soothe sore throats. Kids usually prefer the flavour of oxymels, which are generally more palatable than a straight-up herbal vinegar.

Vinegars & Oxymels in This Book

How to Make a Herbal Vinegar

YOU WILL NEED

Your choice of herbs
Apple cider vinegar (look for a raw organic vinegar)
Clean, dry, wide-mouthed jar with lid
Natural baking parchment
Labels
Muslin (cheesecloth) and fine-mesh strainer

METHOD

1. Half-fill the jar with dried herbs or fill three-quarters if you are using fresh herbs. Pour over the vinegar, making sure all the herbs are covered. Stir well.

2. Place a square of baking parchment over the mouth of the jar and seal with the lid. The baking parchment will stop the vinegar corroding the lid.

3. Label the jar and then allow to infuse for 4 weeks.

4. Strain the vinegar into a jug (pitcher) using a strainer lined with a piece of muslin to remove the herbal material. If using dried herbs, make sure you squeeze out all the goodness from the herbs by wringing the muslin cloth. If using fresh herbs, allow the vinegar to drip through the cloth in its own time so no extra water is introduced into the vinegar from the fresh herbs.

5. Pour the strained vinegar into a clean, dry jar or bottle, seal with the lid and label.

If using fresh herbs, keep the finished herbal vinegar refrigerated and use within 3 months. A herbal vinegar made with dried herbs does not need to be kept in the fridge and will last at least a year.

How to Make an Oxymel

YOU WILL NEED

Your choice of herbs
1 part apple cider vinegar (look for a raw organic vinegar)
1 part raw honey
Clean, dry, wide-mouthed jar with lid
Natural baking parchment
Labels
Muslin (cheesecloth) and fine-mesh strainer

METHOD

1. Follow steps 1–3 for How to Make a Herbal Vinegar, adding equal amounts of honey and vinegar at the same time. Label the jar and then allow to infuse for 4 weeks.

2. Strain the oxymel into a jug (pitcher) using a strainer lined with a piece of muslin to remove the herbal material. Pour the strained oxymel into a clean, dry jar, seal with the lid and label.

The oxymel will last about 3 months if made with fresh herbs or up to a year or longer if made with dried ingredients. If using fresh herbs, store the oxymel in the fridge.

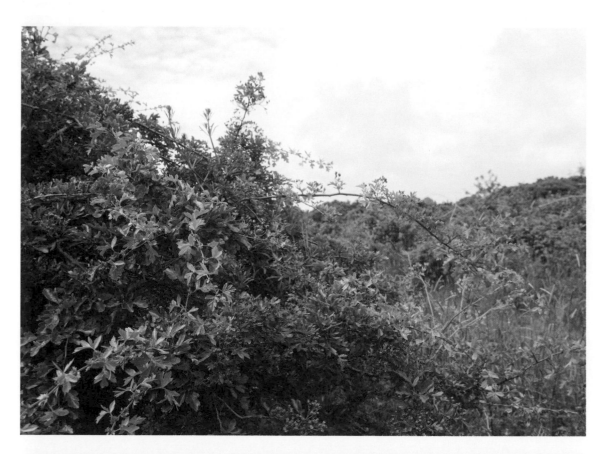

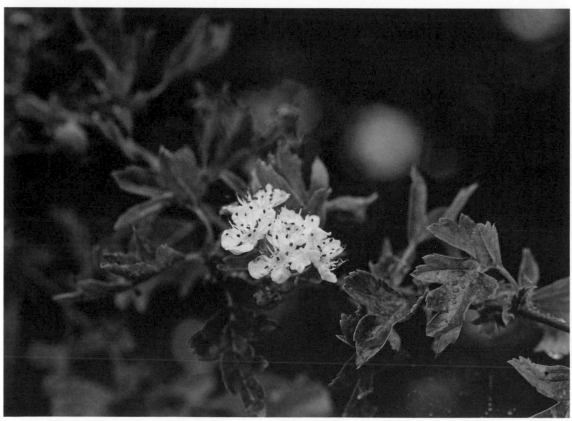

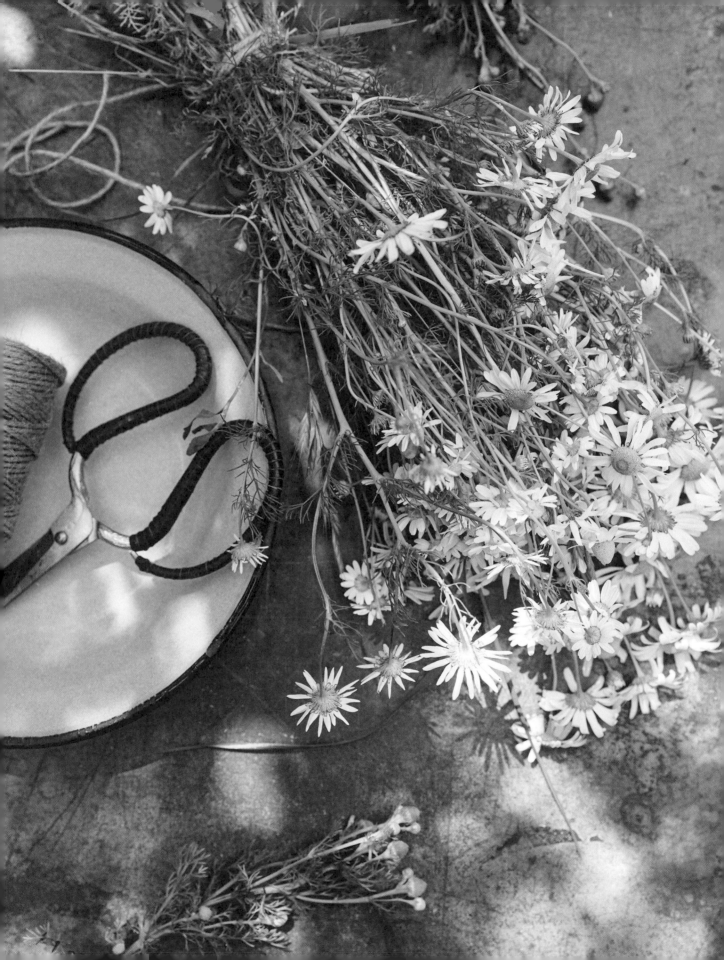

HERBAL HONEYS

Herbal honeys are a combination of herbs and honey that together create a sweet, gentle plant medicine. One of my favourite recipes is for an aromatic rose honey. This sweetly perfumed honey is absolute heaven spooned over a bowl of yoghurt or stirred into herbal teas. It's always something I reach for when I feel myself getting a little blue in the midst of winter. A jar of jewel-coloured, fruity elderberry honey is another favourite and an excellent addition to an elderberry syrup in place of sugar.

Honey is a combination of sugar, pollen, wax and aromatics. It has anti-inflammatory and antibacterial properties in itself, but when combined with herbs it becomes a really special remedy. I always use raw honey where I can because it has far more health benefits and tastes incredible in comparison to big brands of honey. As is the case with most things, honey certainly isn't an endless commodity and so should be used with respect and gratitude and ideally sourced locally. When making herbal honeys with this attitude and a knowledge of where your honey was sourced, then a truly magical remedy can be made.

Of all the solvents (such as water, vinegar and alcohol), honey is the least effective at extracting the medicinal properties from herbs, but there are ways to amp up a herbal honey to make it much stronger. By adding powdered herbs, you can make an electuary which can be taken by the spoon. Or you can just enjoy the sweetness and gentle aromatics of the first method outlined below. Try both and see which you prefer.

Remember: honey should be avoided by children under the age of one.

Herbal Honeys in This Book

Hawthorn Berry Honey (see page 77)
Rose & Lemon Balm Honey (see page 117)

How to Make a Herbal Honey

YOU WILL NEED

Your choice of herbs
Raw honey
Clean, dry, wide-mouthed jar with lid
Label
Fine-mesh strainer (optional)

METHOD

1. If using fresh herbs, chop them up finely, lay out on a lined baking tray (pan) and leave in a warm, dry room overnight or until the herb has wilted and dried out just a little. This reduces the water content and helps preserve the honey for longer. Dried herbs contain no water and so you can omit this step.

2. Add the herbs to the jar until it is one-third full. Pour over the raw honey until the jar is almost full (leave about an inch clear at the top). Stir with a clean, dry wooden chopstick or skewer to combine.

3. Tap the jar firmly on the work surface to knock out any air bubbles. Secure with the lid and label.

4. Leave to infuse in a warm, sunlit area for 4 weeks, stirring with a wooden chopstick/skewer a couple of times throughout this time.

5. Once infused, you can warm the honey very gently in a saucepan, then pour through a strainer to remove the herbs. Alternatively, you can leave the herbs in the honey and consume them together.

6. If you use dried herbs, the honey will last for many years. If using fresh herbs or a juicy herb, such as garlic, keep in the fridge and use within 2 months.

How to Make an Electuary

YOU WILL NEED

Your choice of dried powdered herbs
Raw honey
Small jar with lid
Clean, dry, wide-mouthed jar with lid
Label

METHOD

1. Shake the dried powdered herbs together in a small, dry jar.

2. Pour enough honey into the dried herbs to make a thick paste.

3. Stir the honey and herbs well and cover with a plate or dish towel. Leave the mixture for a day to let it fully infuse and develop. If the mixture is too stiff, add more honey – you want a spreadable texture.

4. Pour the electuary into the wide-mouthed jar, seal with the lid and label. Electuaries will keep for many years.

To use, take 1 teaspoon daily.

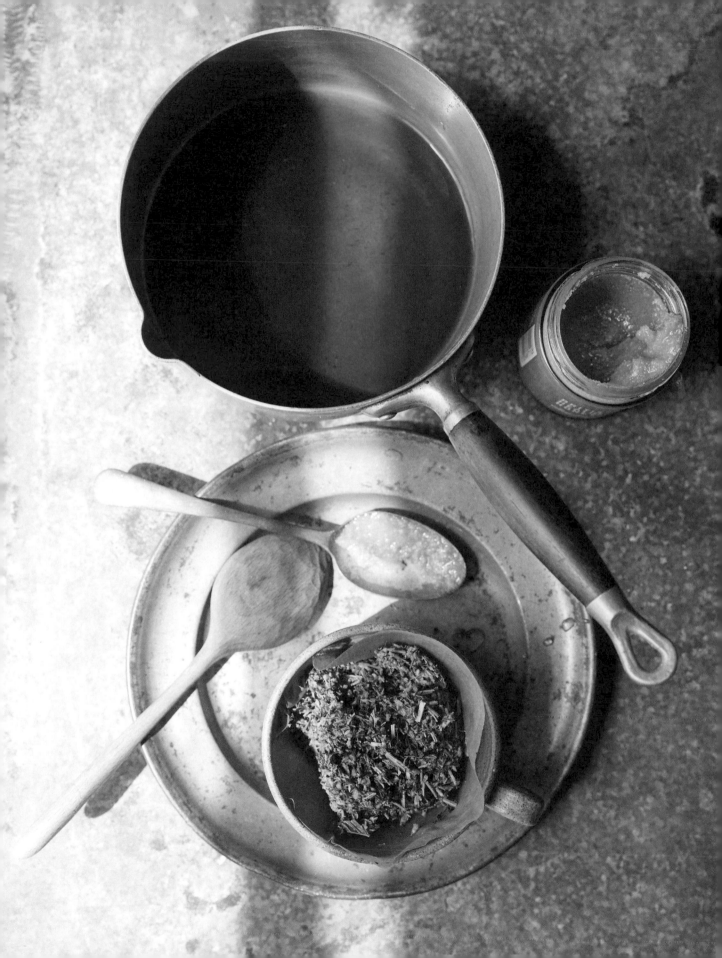

HERBAL SYRUPS

Herbal syrups are very strong herbal teas preserved with sugar. Due to their effectiveness, they are a mainstay of my home apothecary. Elderberry, gently spiced with warming clove and cinnamon, is made every autumn, filling the kitchen with that unmistakable, juicy berry scent. In winter I turn to thyme for the respiratory system and a syrup of yarrow, mint and elderflower for colds and flu. In the warmer seasons I use flower syrups in baking and as cordials and cocktails that are imbued with the very fragrance of a warm sunny day.

Syrups are a deliciously sweet way of taking herbs, thanks to the addition of sugar, honey or maple syrup. I find syrups are a great way of administering herbs to children as the stronger flavour of the herb is made far more palatable with the addition of sugar.

A syrup is made either by creating an infusion or decoction, depending on which parts of the herb you are using. Sugar is then added to preserve the herbal liquid. The more sugar present in the syrup, the more shelf-stable the syrup will be. My favourite way of making a syrup is by using an infused honey, as this way I have an extra dose of herbal power in the end product and a healthier sweetener than refined sugar.

You can add alcohol such as vodka, brandy or even a tincture in order to preserve the syrup further. Herbal syrups need to be kept in the refrigerator and used within weeks or months depending on the sugar quantity and whether alcohol is included.

Syrups in This Book

How to Make a Herbal Syrup

YOU WILL NEED

125 g (4 oz) of your choice of herbs
60–125 g (2–4 oz/½–1 cup) sweetener
375–500 ml (12–16 fl oz/1½–2 cups) water water (depending on whether you use the decoction or infusion method)
1–2 tablespoons tincture or brandy (optional)
Muslin (cheesecloth) and fine-mesh strainer
Storage jar or bottle with lid
Label

METHOD

1. For roots, berries and bark, make the syrup using the decoction method. Add a cup of herbs to a saucepan. Pour over 500 ml (16 fl oz/2 cups) of water and bring to a simmer until about half of the water has evaporated. Strain the liquid into a jug (pitcher) to remove the herbs, wringing out the muslin to get all the liquid from the herbs. Measure out 250 ml (8½ fl oz/1 cup) of the liquid. If you have less than this, add some more water.

2. For the infusion method, which is better suited to more delicate flowers and leaves, boil 375 ml (12 fl oz/1½ cups) of water and pour over 125 g (4 oz) of herbs in a heatproof bowl. Cover and infuse for 1–4 hours. Strain the liquid into a jug, keeping the liquid and discarding the herbs.

3. Pour 250 ml (8½ fl oz/1 cup) of the decocted or infused liquid into a saucepan and add your sweetener. If you are using sugar, stir over a low heat until it has dissolved. If using honey, keep off the heat and stir well until fully incorporated. If you're adding alcohol, do so now.

4. Pour into a clean, dry jar or bottle, seal with the lid and label. Store in the fridge and use within 4 weeks.

For children, take 1 teaspoon; for adults, 1 tablespoon. In acute situations the syrup can be taken up to five times a day. Consult with a clinical herbalist for exact dosage.

INFUSED HERBAL OILS

Infused oils are oils that have been steeped with beneficial herbs. Much like herbal vinegars, infused oils contain some of the herb's properties, making them a useful addition to the home apothecary. I use herbal oils topically, either in salves or balms or directly as a body oil. I also like to make my own culinary oils for cooking.

My favourite topical infused oil is a copper-hued calendula oil. This golden liquid is divine if you get dry, itchy or sore skin and is incredibly gentle, so suits children, too. Once imbued with a few intensely aromatic drops of essential oil you have a luxurious bath oil.

Other favourites of mine are chamomile-infused oil, rosemary oil, and rose, chickweed and lavender infused oil. In general, you will want to use dried herbs to make infused oils. This way, you are introducing the minimum amount of water to your oil, which will prevent spoiling.

There are a handful of herbs that do work better when infused fresh and tend to lose their properties when dried. St John's wort is the main herb in this category. I like to wilt these types of herbs before adding the oil. To do this, I lay the fresh herbs on a baking sheet or tray (pan) and leave them somewhere warm overnight. When wilted, the herbs will have reduced some of their moisture content, helping to keep the oil shelf-stable for longer.

As well as herbs you will need a carrier oil to make an infused oil. A carrier oil is a base oil such as olive oil, sweet almond oil, sunflower or sesame oil. Each carrier oil has its own benefits. My favourite is sunflower oil for topical use as it is affordable and not too strongly scented. For facial application I like to use jojoba oil as it is easily absorbed and is unlikely to block pores.

Culinary infused oils are slightly different in that it is absolutely essential that you use dried herbs. You don't want to consume an oil that has any risk of going bad and by using dried herbs you can be sure that no water is being introduced. I prefer to use a tasty base oil like organic olive oil and like to add deliciously aromatic herbs such as basil, lemon, thyme or rosemary. My method for making a culinary oil is the same as making for a topical herbal oil.

Infused Oils in This Book

Botanical Facial Oil (see page 134)
Chamomile & Oat Bath Melt (see page 71)
Forest Skin Oil (see page 107)
Invigorating Cleavers Massage Oil (see page 83)

How to Make an Infused Oil

YOU WILL NEED

Dried or wilted herb
Carrier oil
Clean, dry, wide-mouthed jar with lid
Labels
Muslin (cheesecloth) and fine-mesh strainer
Storage bottle with lid

METHOD

1. Roughly chop the dried or wilted herbs and place in the jar, filling it roughly half-full.

2. Pour over your choice of carrier oil, filling the jar and making sure all the herbs are covered. Use a clean, dry chopstick to stir and release any air bubbles.

3. Seal the jar with the lid and label, then let the oil infuse for 4 weeks, giving it a little shake every few days or so.

4. When ready, place a strainer lined with a piece of muslin over a jug (pitcher). Pour the oil into the lined strainer. If you are using dried herbs, squeeze the muslin tightly to ensure all the oil has been removed from the herbs. If using wilted herbs, let the oil drip through into the jug, but do not squeeze the cloth.

5. Funnel the infused oil into a clean, dry bottle, seal with a lid and label.

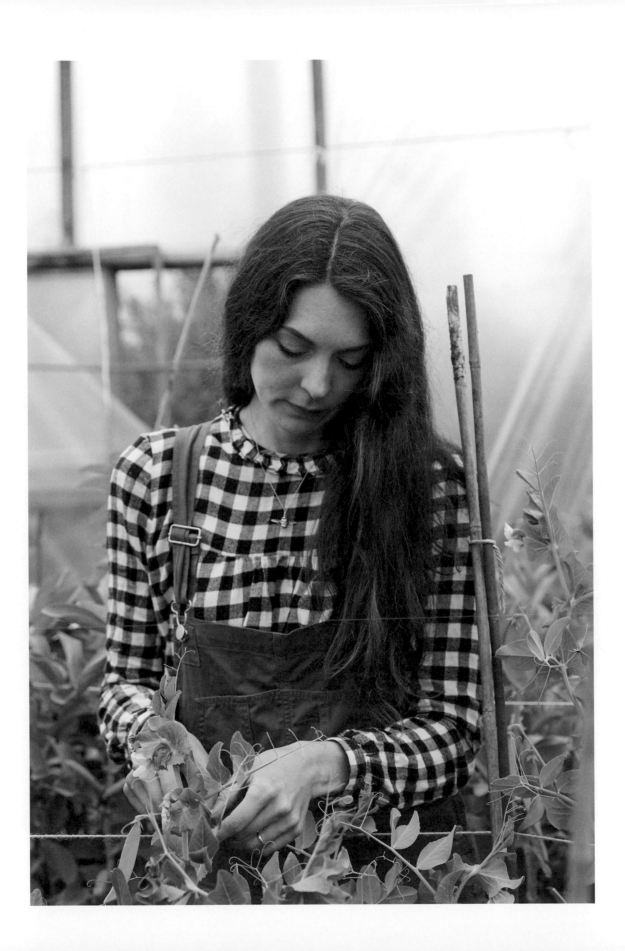

TINCTURES & GLYCERITES

Tinctures are the most potent of the remedies I've listed here and a great way of taking herbs medicinally. Using a strong alcohol, the herbs' properties are extracted into the alcohol and preserved indefinitely.

Tinctures are quick to take, easy to transport and can work relatively quickly in acute situations (such as for insomnia or easing a headache). They are very well suited to our busy lives and definitely worth getting to know.

When choosing the alcohol in which to extract the herbs, I like to find a very high-proof vodka such as an 80 (which is labelled 40% alcohol). Any lower than this will reduce the shelf stability of the tincture. Otherwise, you can use a high-proof brandy or other alcohol if you wish, but bear in mind the shelf life will be shorter.

If you don't like the idea of using alcohol, you can make a glycerite instead. This is the same as a tincture but uses vegetable glycerin instead of alcohol as the base. The glycerin will not do as good a job as alcohol but still makes a very good extraction that is well suited to those avoiding alcohol or for children.

You can make tinctures and glycerites with fresh or dried herbs and can either use single herbs or a combination. When it comes to making a tincture, I prefer to use the folk method. This more traditional method relies on 'eyeballing' the quantities rather than accurately measuring out each ingredient. It is less precise than the measured clinical technique but works beautifully for the gentle herbs mentioned in this book.

Remember that tinctures can be quite powerful remedies, so, if in doubt, work with a clinical herbalist to establish correct dosing and to help you choose the right herbs for you.

Tinctures & Glycerites in This Book

Garden Blossom Glycerite (see page 86)
Healing Herbal Mouthwash (see page 63)
Night-time Glycerite (see page 95)
Rosemary Memory Tincture (see page 125)
Skin Support Tincture (see page 80)
Sage Gargle for Sore Throats (see page 131)

How to Make a Tincture

YOU WILL NEED

Your choice of herbs
Strong vodka or brandy
Clean, dry, wide-mouthed jar with lid
Natural baking parchments
Labels
Muslin (cheesecloth) and fine-mesh strainer
Dropper bottle

METHOD

1. Finely chop the herbs, then add to the jar, making sure this is about half-full if using dried herbs and three-quarters full for fresh herbs.

2. Pour over your choice of alcohol, filling the jar and covering all of the plant matter. Stir with a clean, dry wooden skewer or chopstick to remove any air bubbles.

3. Place a square of baking parchment over the mouth of the jar, seal with the lid and label. The baking parchment will stop the lid from corroding.

4. Keep the jar in a dark, dry place to infuse for about 4–6 weeks, giving it a shake and some good intentions when you remember.

5. When the tincture is ready, strain into a jug (pitcher) using a strainer lined with a piece of muslin to remove the herbs. Wring out all the liquid from the muslin. Funnel this strained liquid into a clean, dry dropper bottle and label. Any excess tincture can be stored in a lidded bottle until needed. There is no shelf life for an alcohol tincture made with dried herbs, but discard it in the unlikely event that it grows mould or begins to ferment.

The dose for adults is approx. 1–3 teaspoons per day. I like to take mine diluted in some water.

How to Make a Glycerite

YOU WILL NEED

Your choice of herbs
Vegetable glycerin (ensure it is food-safe)
Clean, dry, wide-mouthed jar with lid
Labels
Muslin (cheesecloth) and fine-mesh strainer
Dropper bottle

METHOD

1. Half-fill the jar with dried herbs or fill until three-quarters full if using fresh herbs. Pour over the glycerin, filling the jar and covering all of the plant matter. If you are using dried herbs, dilute the glycerin with water – mixing 3 parts glycerin to 1 part water. Stir with a clean, dry wooden skewer or chopstick to remove any air bubbles.

2. Seal the jar with the lid and label. Store in a dark, dry place to infuse for about 4–6 weeks, giving the jar a shake as for the standard tincture method.

3. When the infusion is ready, strain the glycerite into a jug (pitcher) using a strainer lined with a piece of muslin to remove the herbs. Wring out all the liquid from the cloth.

4. Funnel the strained liquid into a clean, dry dropper bottle, then label.

Glycerites have a shelf life of 1–2 years.

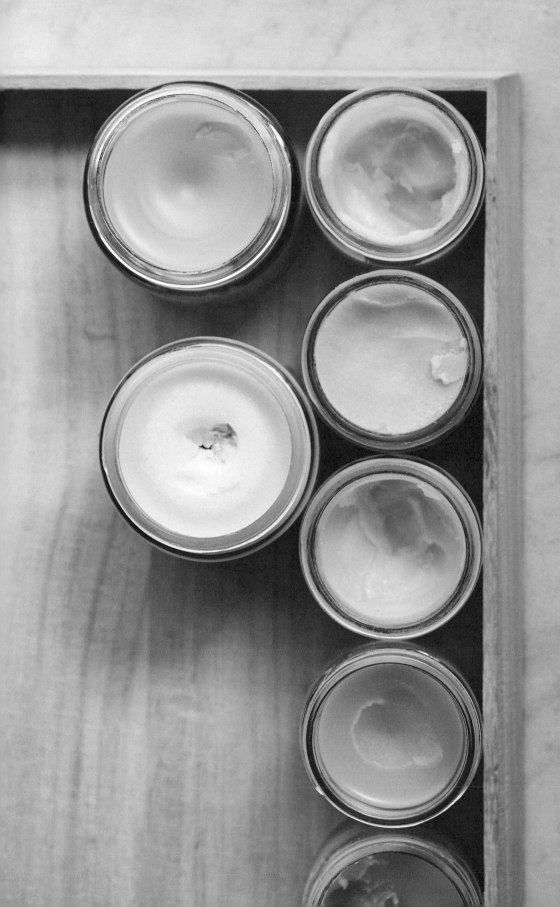

SALVES & BALMS

Creating salves and balms from scratch means saying goodbye to the questionable ingredients and preservatives you find in most store-bought products. It gives you total control and the ability to concoct exquisite bespoke skincare products.

Salves are a combination of wax and herbal oil (and often aromatic essential oils) that have a solid texture. Depending on what oils you use, they are great for dealing with small areas of the skin that need some extra care, such as a graze or patch of sore skin, for soothing headaches and achy joints, and dabbing on the temples or pulse points for a mood booster. The wax in the salve acts as a protective barrier, too.

Salves aren't suitable for use on fresh burns or on any weepy skin as they will trap in moisture and heat.

Essential oils are a wonderful addition to salves and can really help boost their effects. In general, a 2–5% dilution of essential oils is used in salves, but if using them on children, make sure you use a safe dilution such as 0.5% or 1%. See the Essential Oil Dilution Chart on page 51 for more details on using essential oils in salves and balms.

Balms are similar to salves, containing herbal oils and beeswax, but they have more of a buttery texture due to the addition of plant butters, such as shea or cocoa butter. Balms are used on larger areas, such as the hands, or as a full body balm. They are very softening and wonderful for treating dry skin or soothing sore, garden-weary hands. The plant butters have their own properties, too. For example, unrefined cocoa butter has a chocolatey scent and high vitamin E content, while rose hip seed butter is excellent for older skin.

The lack of water in both balms and salves means they have a long shelf life. They are also easy to make.

Salves & Balms in This Book

Gardener's Ointment for Sore Joints & Muscles (see page 126)
Gentle Chickweed & Borage Balm (see page 140)
Lemon Balm for the Lips (see page 93)
Plantain & Daisy Bruise Salve (see page 112)
Tension Relief Balm (see page 100)
Veg Plot Hand Balm with Carrot & Calendula (see page 64)

How to Make a Salve

YOU WILL NEED

3 tablespoons herbal-infused oil
1½ teaspoons beeswax pellets
Essential oils, if desired, at the correct dilution
  (see the Essential Oil Dilution Chart opposite)
Double boiler
Wide-mouthed jar or tin with lid
Label

METHOD

1. Add the herbal oil and beeswax to a double boiler. Let the beeswax melt into the herbal oil over a low heat.

2. Remove from the heat and stir in the essential oils (if using). Please note: It is common to use a higher percentage (around 3–5%) of essential oils when making salves.

3. Pour the mixture into the jar or tin, seal with the lid and label. Let the salve set for 24 hours before using.

The salve should last up to one year.

How to Make a Balm

YOU WILL NEED

3 tablespoons herbal-infused oil
1 tablespoon beeswax pellets
85 g (3 oz) shea butter, roughly chopped
Essential oils, if desired, at the correct dilution
  (see the Essential Oil Dilution Chart opposite)
Double boiler
Small jar or tin with lid
Label

METHOD

1. Add the herbal oil and beeswax to a double boiler and warm very gently over a low heat until the wax begins to melt.

2. Add the shea butter and gently melt. Add the essential oils (if using) and stir.

3. Pour the mixture into the jar or tin, seal with the lid and label. Allow the balm to cool and set for 24 hours before using.

The balm should last up to one year.

Essential Oil Dilution Chart

This chart will give you a good starting point for using essential oils safely in any homemade, topical recipe. Essential oils are incredibly potent and a little goes a long way. If in doubt, use less to start with and see how you get on. A 5% dilution is great for salves where only a small amount of product is used and in acute situations, but this won't be suitable for children or for those with sensitive skin.

Example: If I was making a salve using 50 ml (1¾ fl oz/3 tablespoons) of infused oil, I would add 75 drops of essential oil for a 5% dilution. If you are looking for more information, I highly recommend Robert Tisserand and Rodney Young's book Essential Oil Safety.

Carrier Oil	0.5%	1%	2%	3%	5%
10 ml (2 teaspoons)	1 drop	3 drops	6 drops	9 drops	15 drops
15 ml (1 tablespoon)	2 drops	4 drops	9 drops	13 drops	22 drops
30 ml (2 tablespoons)	4 drops	9 drops	18 drops	27 drops	45 drops
50 ml (3 tablespoons)	7 drops	15 drops	30 drops	45 drops	75 drops

Suitable Dilution Levels

The quantity of essential oil you add depends on how you plan to use the remedy and the age of the person being treated. The following dilution levels are recommended:

0.5%	Babies over the age of 6 months (although you should only use suitable essential oils such as lavender) as well as the elderly or people with compromised immune systems.
1%	Children over 2 years as well as pregnant or frail people. Use for facial products.
2–3%	Use for body and bath products. For the nervous system and emotions.
5%	For salves, specific and acute problems, and short-term use.

Chapter Four

Plant Profiles

Now that you know the basic herbalist techniques it's time to put them to the test. Gather up your garden trug and let's explore the common garden herbs that can be turned into herbal medicine.

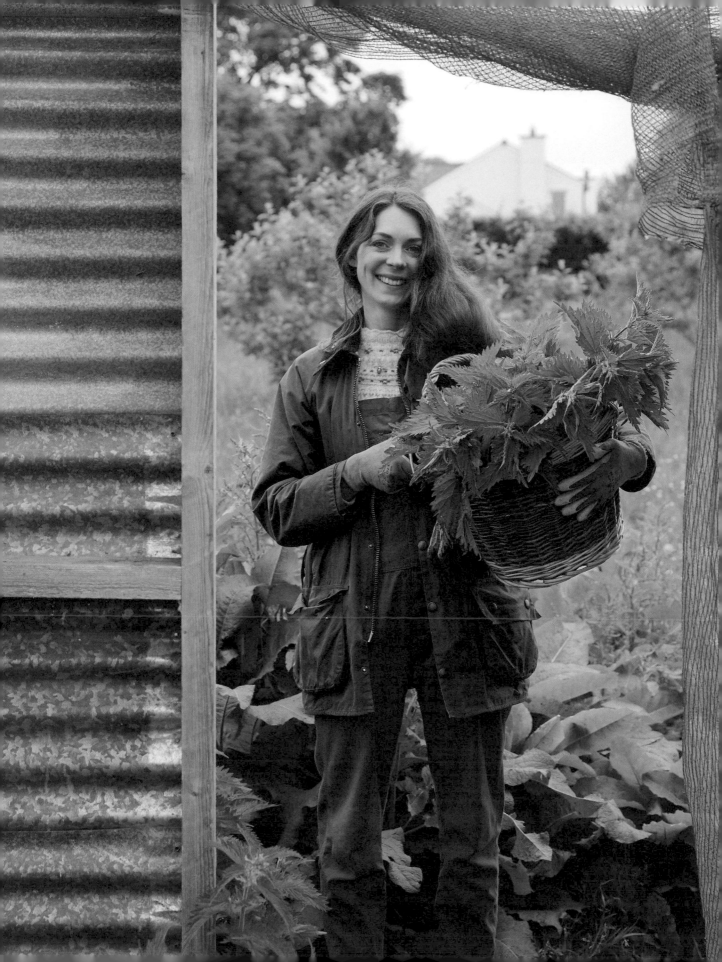

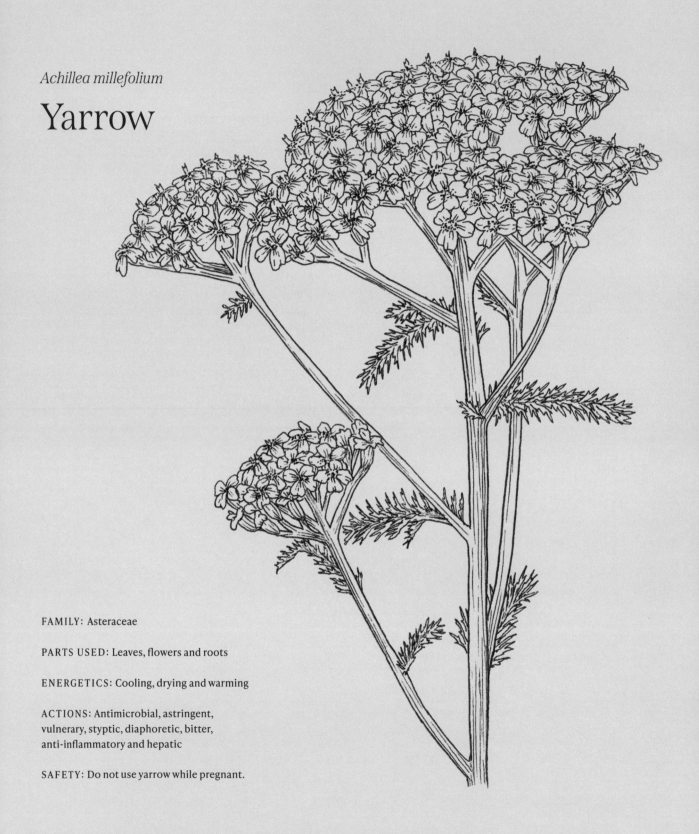

Achillea millefolium

Yarrow

FAMILY: Asteraceae

PARTS USED: Leaves, flowers and roots

ENERGETICS: Cooling, drying and warming

ACTIONS: Antimicrobial, astringent, vulnerary, styptic, diaphoretic, bitter, anti-inflammatory and hepatic

SAFETY: Do not use yarrow while pregnant.

Over the years I've gotten to know my patch of wild yarrow well. Growing in a bunch under an elder tree, its pretty white flowers bob about all summer long and even through most of winter I can find its beautiful feathery leaves hiding amongst the tired brown grass.

I usually harvest yarrow in a rush. As the mother of two toddlers, I know I can grab a small handful of this plant and make a quick poultice to ease childhood grazes and cuts. You'll often find me crouched down by a patch of yarrow, disgruntled toddler in one arm and a bunch of yarrow in the other, as I gently work with its potent antimicrobial and healing qualities to soothe scratches and cuts.

IDENTIFICATION

Yarrow has very distinctive leaves, which are divided deeply and sit alternately on the stem. Its flowers are creamy white and look a little like tiny daisies. The stem is coated in tiny hairs and is slightly woody when snapped.

USES

It's not surprising that yarrow has also been called woundwort or carpenter's weed. Its antimicrobial and wound-healing abilities have made it a useful herb for many generations. It's at its most potent and powerful used fresh from the plant and I recommend you try using it as a poultice. It's also often recommended for itchy skin and rashes.

Yarrow is a styptic. This simply means that the herb has the ability to slow and staunch blood flow when the plant is applied to the affected area. Along with its antimicrobial qualities, this makes yarrow an important herb to grow and learn to use. Next time you need to deal with a cut or scrape, try my Styptic Powder recipe (see page 56) or make a simple yarrow poultice and see it work for yourself!

Yarrow is often associated with women's health and with menstruation in particular. Yarrow can help with heavy or scanty bleeding during menstruation as well as encouraging a more regular cycle.

Yarrow is well known as a herb for fevers and flu. By dilating capillaries, it helps to break and cool a fever. It's one of my favourite herbs to reach for if I feel a cold coming on, especially when combined with peppermint and elderflower.

It's common to find yarrow as an ingredient in herbal bitters. Bitters are a combination of digestive and bitter-tasting herbs that are infused into alcohol and usually consumed as drops before a meal to help stimulate the digestive system. Yarrow, with its carminative effects and bitter flavour, is a great addition to homemade bitters.

HARVESTING & PREPARATION

Harvest the long stems of flowering yarrow and hang them in bunches to dry. Otherwise, remove the flowers and the leaves and lay on a drying tray in a warm, airy room or in a food dehydrator set at 42°C (108°F). The dried flowers and leaves can be stored in an airtight jar for at least 12 months.

Styptic Powder

Yarrow, with its ability to staunch bleeding, is a must-have in a first aid kit. This powder is perfect for sprinkling over fresh cuts and minor wounds where you want to slow down and stop bleeding. Its antiseptic and antimicrobial qualities are also wonderful at helping to keep the area clean. Keep a jar of this powder with you at all times!

YOU WILL NEED

Dried yarrow leaves and flowers
High speed coffee blender
Small tin or jar
Label

METHOD

Sort through the leaves and flowers, ensuring there are no stalks. Blitz them in a coffee blender until a fine powder has formed.

Let the powder settle before opening the blender and then pour into a jar or tin.

Label with the contents and date.

TO USE

Use a small pinch to help stop bleeding of minor cuts or wounds. Ideally, clean the area well before use. An alternative to this powder is to create a yarrow tincture and use a drop of this for a similar effect. See page 47 for guidance on how to make a tincture.

Gypsy Cold & Flu Syrup

The combination of these three herbs is a true classic and one that most herbalists will know very well! Said to be derived from a traditional gypsy recipe, this blend can help break a fever and support immunity during colds and flus.

YOU WILL NEED

40 g (1½ oz/⅓ cup) dried elderflower
40 g (1½ oz/⅓ cup) dried yarrow leaves
40 g (1½ oz/⅓ cup) dried peppermint leaves
375 ml (12 fl oz/1½ cups) boiling water
62–125 g (2¼ oz–4 oz/½–1 cup) honey or sugar
Heatproof bowl
Muslin (cheesecloth) and fine-mesh strainer
Storage bottle with lid

METHOD

Place all the dried herbs in a heatproof bowl and pour over the boiling water. Leave to infuse for 1–4 hours.

Strain the liquid into a jug (pitcher) using a sieve and muslin cloth to remove the herbs. Measure out 250 ml (8½ fl oz/1 cup) of herbal liquid.

Pour the liquid into a saucepan and add the honey or sugar. Gently warm to combine. If using sugar, ensure that all the sugar has completely dissolved before removing from the heat. Funnel into a bottle and label. Keep refrigerated and use within a few weeks.

TO USE

Take up to 1 tablespoon three to five times a day during acute situations.

This syrup is not suitable for pregnant or nursing mothers.

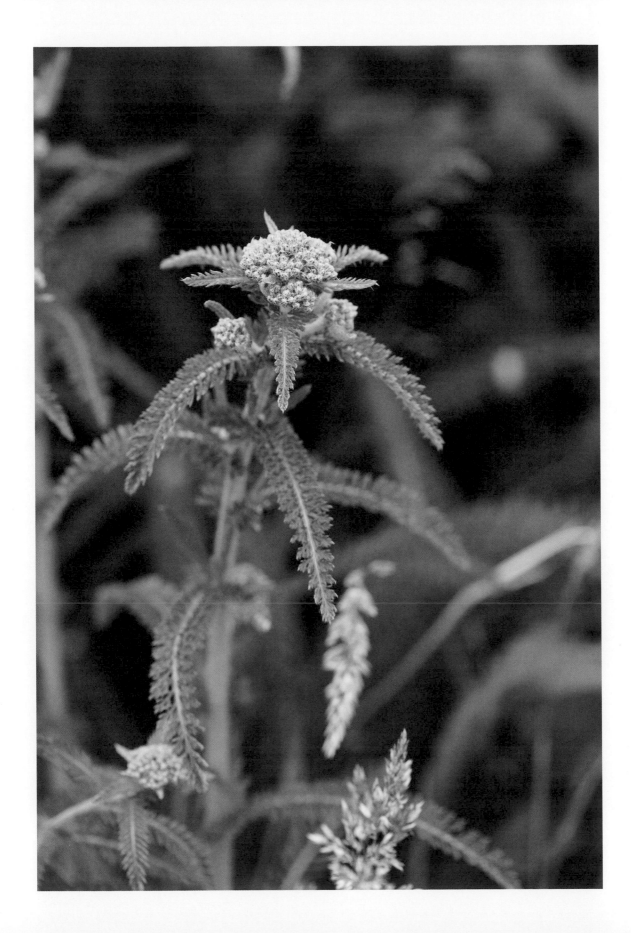

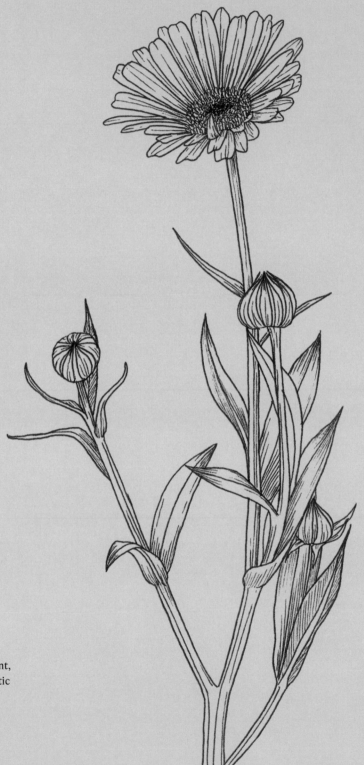

Calendula officinalis

Calendula

FAMILY: Asteraceae

PARTS USED: Flowers

ENERGETICS: Neutral

ACTIONS: Anti-inflammatory, antispasmodic, anti-fungal, astringent, cholagogue, emmenagogue, lymphatic and vulnerary

SAFETY: Avoid if allergic to members of the Asteraceae family and during pregnancy.

With its bright, sunny flowers, sticky texture and pine-like scent, calendula is a must-have in my garden. Here in Northern Ireland my calendula plants happily flower well into late autumn and one of my favourite moments in spring is planting their little curled seeds ready for a new season in the garden.

Calendula is a hard-working plant. Not only do its orange flowers brighten up garden beds and containers and lure aphids away from other plants, but its bright petals are also edible and make a great addition to salads, bakes and stews (a traditional favourite). More importantly, however, the whole flower, including its green calyx, is full of powerful plant medicine that can be harnessed in many ways.

Personally, I take such joy in filling my big glass apothecary jars with the dried but still vibrant flowers. I store these on my shelves alongside other dried garden flowers like chamomile and rose. Even a glimpse of these stored blooms on a dreary winter's day brings a smile to my face.

IDENTIFICATION

Calendula can be identified by its large, single or double, daisy-shaped flowers in shades of yellow or orange. It has a hairy stem and oblong, alternate leaves.

USES

Calendula is a well-known lymphatic herb. This is the plant to reach for when you find yourself with swollen lymph glands, regular infections and general lymphatic congestion. It gently but effectively encourages lymphatic movement, which in turn helps to promote a healthy immune system and shift toxins. This lymphatic action is also good for helping to clear the skin of acne and other chronic skin conditions. Try a regular full-body massage with a calendula-infused oil to reap the benefits of this plant and also to stimulate the lymph system.

Calendula is also an antifungal and can be used in salves and balms to help rid the skin of mild rashes. Internally, a strong tea is a traditional remedy for fungal infections. You can make a tea with calendula, which can be used as a gargle to help heal mouth ulcers, support gum health and for oral thrush.

Calendula's anti-inflammatory and mildly antimicrobial effects make it a first-rate herb for the skin. This is a plant I often reach for to help support my children's skin. It works beautifully combined with chamomile in nappy creams and as a cradle cap oil (thanks again to its antifungal action) or as a gentle, soothing bedtime balm. If you're prone to eczema, psoriasis or irritated skin, calendula is going to be a sure friend. Calendula is also a great addition to any salve to soothe minor wounds, aiding healing and helping to reduce scarring.

Another wonderful use for calendula is to improve the digestive system. Its anti-inflammatory and astringent actions can help with gastrointestinal issues such as gastric ulcers. Try a blend of equal parts of dried calendula, chamomile, peppermint and marshmallow root for a soothing gut tea.

Calendula's emmenagogue actions can help with delayed and painful menstruation. Try it in a tea or tincture or make a balm with an infused calendula and yarrow oil and add supportive essential oils such as peppermint, yarrow and chamomile, which can be massaged onto the lower abdomen to relieve cramping.

HARVESTING & PREPARATION

The key to a great calendula harvest is to pick the flower heads often (also ensuring you pick the green calyx alongside the flower, as this contains valuable properties). Regular harvesting keeps the plant blooming for a longer period. Once picked, make sure you dry the flowers thoroughly and gently check the centres for any retained moisture. The flower should feel completely crisp and dry. Any moisture can make the flowers go mouldy in the storage jar.

Equinox Tea

This tea blend is the perfect way to welcome in the changing seasons and is particularly suited to the autumnal months when the weather becomes colder and our immunity may be challenged. Calendula and elderberry provide support for the immune system, while rose hip supplies a kick of vitamin C. Cinnamon and ginger give this tea a delicious flavour as well as gently heating the system and aiding circulation.

YOU WILL NEED

1 teaspoon dried elderberries
½ teaspoon dried calendula flowers
1 teaspoon dried rose hip shells (with seeds and hairs removed prior to drying)
Cinnamon stick
¼–2 teaspoons diced fresh ginger root
1 teaspoon hawthorn or plain honey (optional)
Boiling water
Tea strainer

METHOD

Add the elderberries, calendula flowers and rose hip shells to a tea strainer. Crumble in a quarter of the cinnamon stick and add the fresh ginger to taste.

Pour over freshly boiled water into a mug and allow the tea to infuse for 10 minutes.

For some grounding sweetness and heart health protection, you can also stir in some Hawthorn Berry Honey (see page 77).

Try a Tea Ritual

Practise this tea ritual to bring more connection to the herb you are using and to cultivate a sense of gratitude for what you have in front of you in the moment.

Prepare your tea and sit in a comfortable place. Take a moment to feel the warm cup in your hand and smell the tea's scent. Notice the colour of the tea, the scent, the heat. Feel gratitude for this moment. Now take a small sip of tea. Really taste the flavours, notice the warmth and feel the process of lifting the cup to your mouth. Is the herb sweet, bitter? Try and notice as many flavours as you can.

When finished, wash and put away your cup and tea-making utensils thoughtfully and with gratitude.

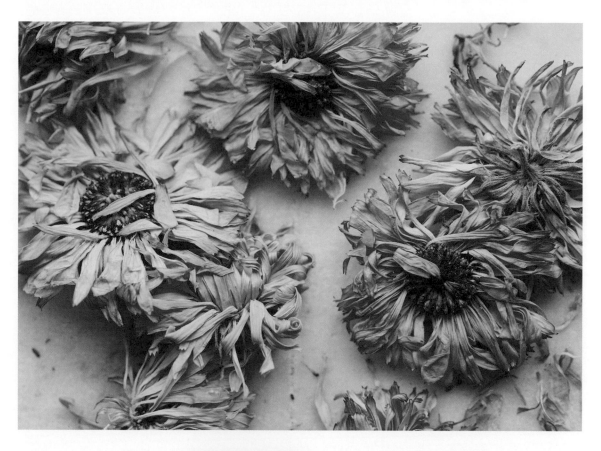

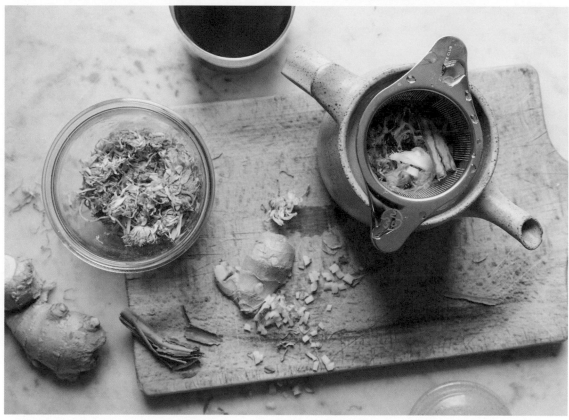

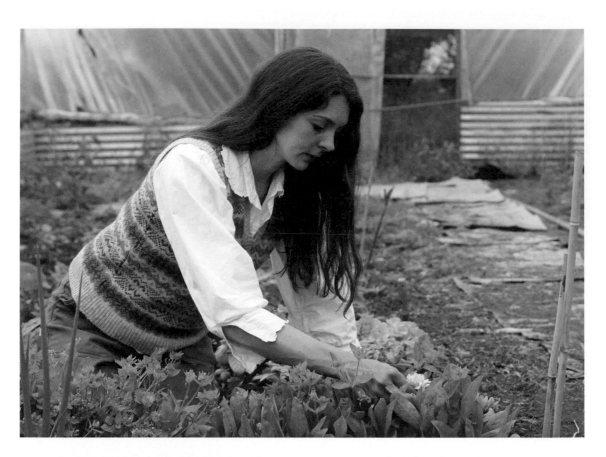

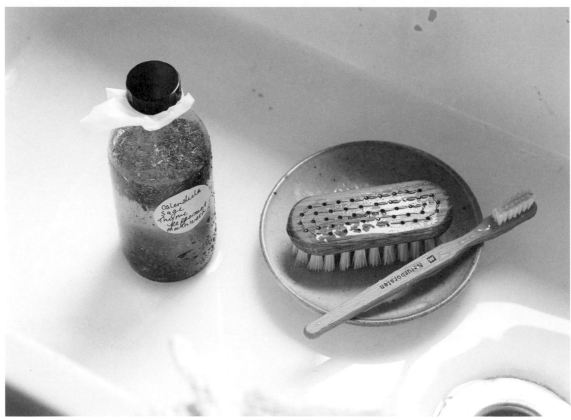

Healing Herbal Mouthwash

If you suffer from mouth ulcers, then this natural mouthwash is for you. This simple and home-grown remedy uses powerful calendula with its affinity for soothing and healing ulcers and gums, as well as thyme, sage and peppermint.

YOU WILL NEED

1 part dried calendula flower
1 part dried sage leaf
1 part dried thyme leaf
1 part dried peppermint leaf
Vodka
Clean, dry, wide-mouthed jar with lid
Natural baking parchment
Labels
Muslin (cheesecloth) and fine mesh strainer
Glass storage bottle with lid

METHOD

Half-fill the jar with all the herbs. I use equals parts of each herb in this recipe and 'eyeball' the quantities as I add them to the jar, as opposed to using weighing scales.

Once you have added the herbs to the jar, pour over the vodka until the plant material is completely covered. Give everything a good mix, ensuring all the plant matter is well coated in vodka. Pour in more vodka if necessary.

Place a square of baking parchment over the top of the jar, seal with the lid and label and date the jar.

Store the jar in a cupboard or anywhere out of direct sunlight and let the combination of vodka and herbs infuse for 4–6 weeks. This ensures the herbs are fully infused into the alcohol. Check your tincture during the first week and add more vodka if needed, as the dry herbs will absorb some of the liquid.

Once the infusion time is over, strain off the plant material using a strainer lined with a piece of muslin. Make sure you squeeze out all of the liquid from the herbal matter. The spent herbs can now be composted.

Use a funnel to transfer the strained tincture to a dry amber glass bottle and label. The tincture will last at least 12 months.

TO USE

To make the mouthwash, add 1 teaspoon of the tincture to a small glass of water. Take a sip and gargle well, then spit out, just as you would with any mouthwash. Use this mouthwash daily in the morning and last thing at night after brushing your teeth. Make up a fresh batch of the mouthwash daily.

Veg Plot Hand Balm with Carrot & Calendula

Whether it's tackling weeds, digging up potatoes or planting, the work on the veg plot inevitably leaves my hands looking and feeling worse for wear. For thorns and scratches, as well as general wear and tear, a good hand cream is essential. This rich balm contains our hero plant calendula with its anti-inflammatory properties, as well as lavender for antibacterial and healing support and carrot seed essential oil for extra anti-inflammatory qualities. It also contains shea butter which nourishes hardworking hands.

YOU WILL NEED

1 tablespoon beeswax pellets
2 tablespoons calendula-infused sunflower oil
   (see page 44 for how to make an infused herbal oil)
1 tablespoon carrot-infused oil)
85 g (3 oz) shea butter, roughly chopped
5 drops lavender essential oil
5 drops carrot seed essential oil
Double boiler
Small jar or tin with lid
Label

METHOD

Melt the beeswax in a double boiler. Once melted, pour in the calendula- and carrot-infused oils and add the shea butter. Stir gently until the butter has just melted.

Remove from the heat and dry off the base of the pan. Add the essential oils and stir.

Pour the liquid balm into the jar or tin and place in the fridge to set. Once cooled and set, label.

The balm will last 12 months.

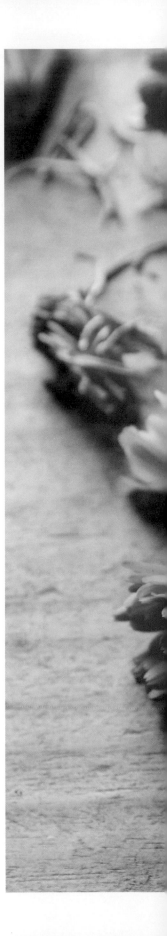

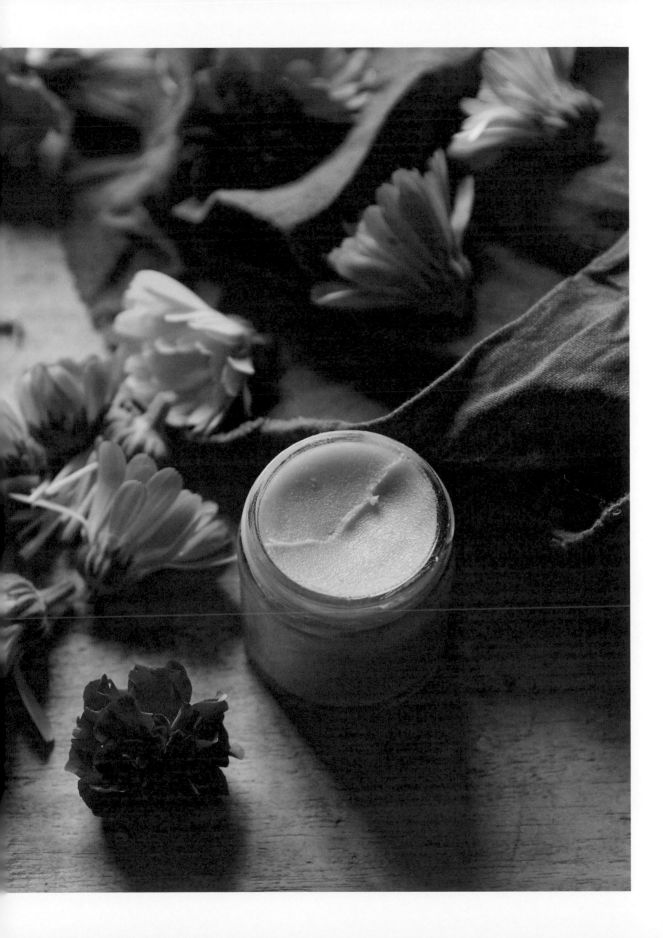

Chamaemelum nobile
& Matricaria chamomilla

Chamomile

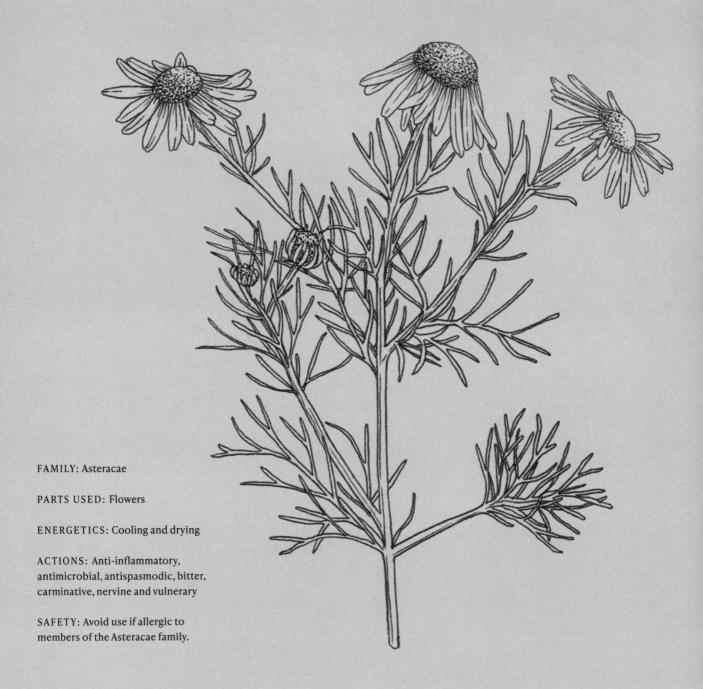

FAMILY: Asteracae

PARTS USED: Flowers

ENERGETICS: Cooling and drying

ACTIONS: Anti-inflammatory,
antimicrobial, antispasmodic, bitter,
carminative, nervine and vulnerary

SAFETY: Avoid use if allergic to
members of the Asteracae family.

One of my first experiences of using herbs medicinally was with chamomile. A couple of dusty teabags lived at the back of our cupboard and would be pulled out as a last resort to induce sleep. I never really gave chamomile much more thought until I began to grow it myself from seed.

Freshly grown chamomile is a world apart from those old teabags! Verdant, fresh and with an apple-like scent, chamomile is one herb that we should all grow.

Pretty to look at with its daisy-like flowers, it takes little effort to grow chamomile and is foolproof to look after once established. A summer's worth of blossom, dried, can fill up quite a few jars and keep you going through the colder seasons.

IDENTIFICATION

Chamomile looks quite similar to a daisy. The white-petalled flowers have a bright yellow centre and sit on a long stem. The leaves are feathery in appearance and pinnate. There is another plant that's similar to chamomile called pineapple weed (*Matricaria discoidea*). This is actually a chamomile too but is usually found growing in the wild. It has a protruding, domed, yellow centre and almost unnoticeable petals and feathery leaves. It grows close to the ground and loves pavements and well-worn, compacted areas. Pineapple weed smells similar to chamomile but with a beautiful pineapple edge and has similar relaxing properties.

USES

Chamomile is well known as a herb that has an affinity with sleep. As a nervine it works beautifully to calm anxiety and is a great herb to drink in a tea before bed – it works equally well for overexcited children as well as overworked and worn-out adults! Chamomile helps to relax the peripheral nerves as well as muscles, which has an overall calming effect on the entire body along with the mind. Try brewing a mug of Chamomile Moon Milk (see page 69) to experience the effects of this soporific and reassuring herb. To calm babies that are fussy due to teething, try saturating a fabric teether or muslin (cheesecloth) in cooled chamomile tea and freeze it for a natural remedy for sore gums.

Chamomile is also an excellent remedy for upset tummies. Its antispasmodic, anti-inflammatory and antimicrobial properties are all great at helping to soothe intestinal walls and ease gas and indigestion. A cup of strong chamomile tea can be sipped throughout the day to calm and hydrate the system. You could also combine a few drops of chamomile essential oil in a carrier oil of choice and massage onto the tummy for relief. For a cramping tummy, try a warm external compress using a strong chamomile tea.

Personally, one of my favourite ways to use chamomile is in skincare. As part of a family prone to dry skin, I use chamomile daily for its calming and anti-inflammatory properties. I also use it on my young children to clear rashes and soothe sensitive skin. I love to make an infused oil from the dried flowers and use this as the base for many skincare products. A bath combining soothing chamomile and oats in a base of nourishing cocoa butter is great for sore and parched skin. See my recipe for Chamomile & Oat Bath Melt on page 71.

Finally, chamomile is a lovely herb to reach for to ease stuffed-up sinuses and congestion, as the anti-catarrhal properties can help to release the build-up of mucus. Try the flowers steeped in a tea or use them in a steam inhalation by pouring boiling water into a basin and adding a handful of chamomile. Once the water is cool enough to be comfortable, lower your head over the basin (covered with a towel) and take deep breaths.

HARVESTING & PREPARATION

Chamomile flowers are ready for harvest in mid-summer. Harvest the flowers on a dry morning when they are open. Pick the heads off the flowers and arrange on a tray in a warm, dry place inside or, alternatively, use a food dehydrator set at around 37°C (99°F).

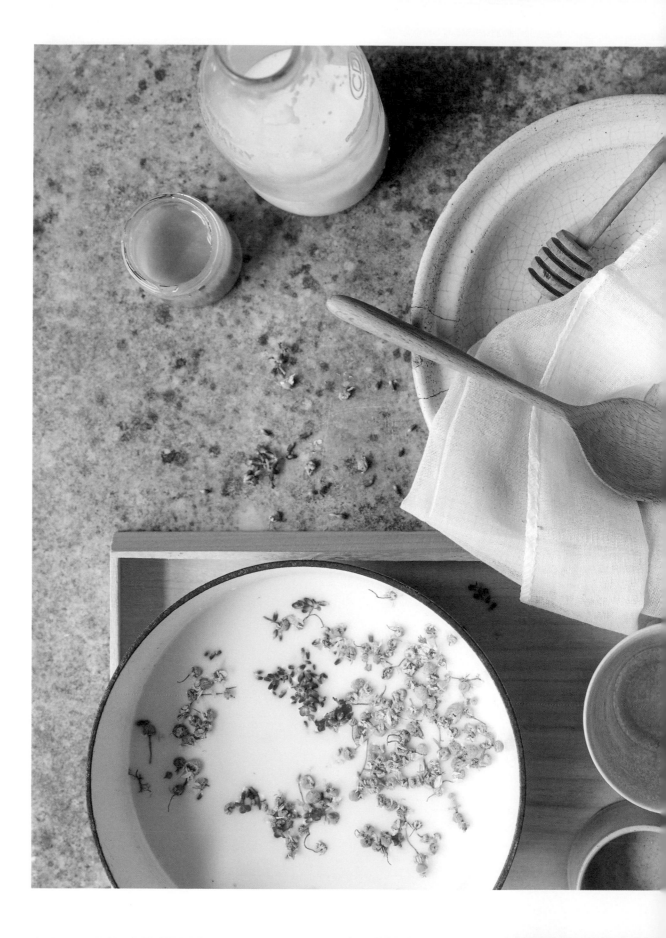

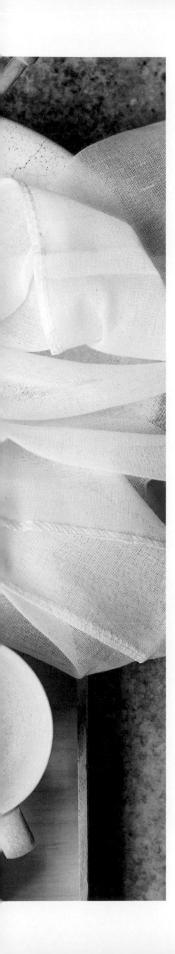

Chamomile Moon Milk

When the night rolls in and it is finally time to put my feet up and grab a book, I love nothing more than a cup of this calming and relaxing moon milk. The gentle ritual of warming the milk with these calming herbs and pouring it into my favourite ceramic mug is a beautiful reminder to my body that the day is complete. With its creamy flavour, this milk is grounding and settling for the nervous system and the combination of chamomile and lavender, two gentle but powerful nervines, helps to ease away any lingering worries and usher in a deep, restorative sleep.

YOU WILL NEED

1 mug of oat or whole milk
2 teaspoons dried or fresh chamomile flowers
Pinch of dried or fresh lavender flowers
1 teaspoon local honey or maple syrup
Tea strainer

METHOD

Pour the milk into a small saucepan and sprinkle in the chamomile and lavender. Make sure you don't add more than a pinch of lavender as it is a strong-tasting herb and can easily overwhelm the moon milk if too much is used.

Gently warm the milk and herbs for around 5 minutes, making sure you don't boil the milk.

After 5 minutes strain the milk into your mug using a tea strainer. Sweeten with the honey or maple syrup, or even better stir in a teaspoon of Rose & Lemon Balm Honey (see page 117).

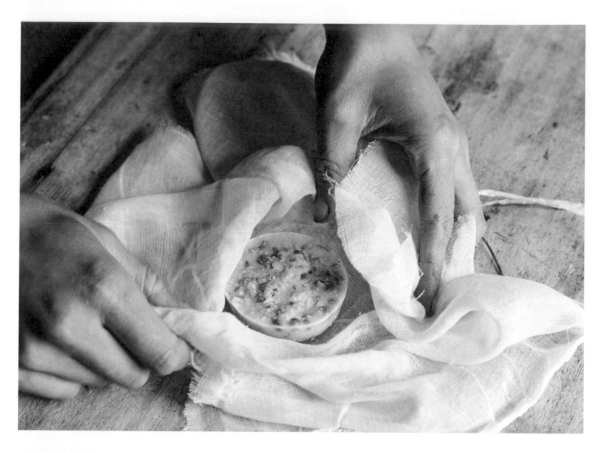

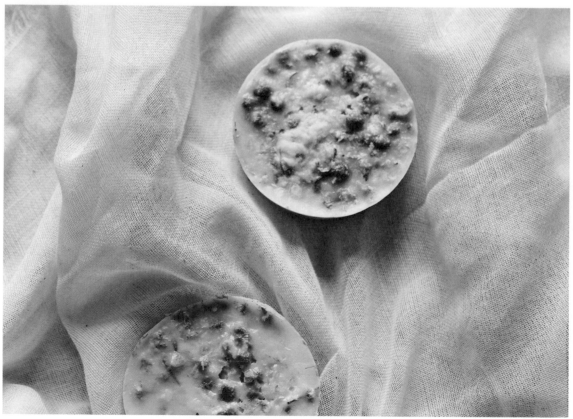

Chamomile & Oat Bath Melt

These bath melts are a complete luxury for itchy, sore skin or those who suffer from eczema. The chamomile flowers create a beautiful bath infusion that treats skin complaints while the oats are soothing and calming to the epidermis. Once made, the bath melts will last about six months in a dry, airtight container.

YOU WILL NEED

1 tablespoon rolled oats
1 tablespoon dried chamomile flowers
70 g (2½ oz) cocoa butter
1½ tablespoons chamomile and calendula-infused sunflower oil
  (see page 44 for how to make an infused herbal oil)
10 drops lavender essential oil
8 drops mandarin essential oil
Small silicon cupcake mould
Double boiler or thick-bottomed saucepan
Muslin (cheesecloth)
Raffia twine

METHOD

Combine the oats and chamomile flowers in a clean, dry bowl. Sprinkle into the silicon moulds, filling these until they are about half-full.

Melt the cocoa butter in a double boiler or saucepan over a low heat. Once melted, add the infused sunflower oil and essential oils, and stir well. Pour the mixture into the filled moulds until you reach the top. Allow to cool overnight.

Once the bath melts are completely hard, pop them out of the moulds, wrap each one in a small square of muslin and secure in place with some raffia twine.

TO USE

Place the bath melt in a warm bath and let it dissolve gradually to create a soothing, milky bath, fragrant with calming oils and herbs. The leftover herbs and oats in the cloth create a sort of bath teabag, infusing the water further with skin-nourishing benefits.

Variations

You can adjust this recipe to make many variations. Try infusing the sunflower oil with rose and lavender instead, swap out the chamomile flowers for rose petals and omit the mandarin oil for a bath melt that will bring back memories of summer.

Crataegus spp.

Hawthorn

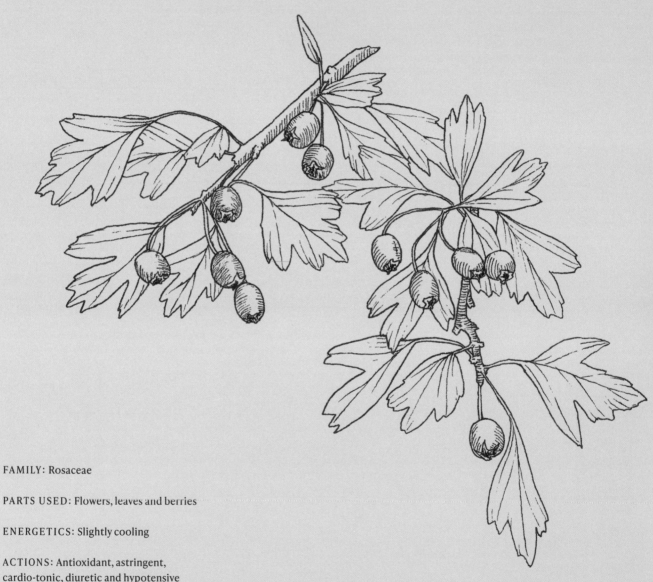

FAMILY: Rosaceae

PARTS USED: Flowers, leaves and berries

ENERGETICS: Slightly cooling

ACTIONS: Antioxidant, astringent,
cardio-tonic, diuretic and hypotensive

SAFETY: Consult a medical professional
if you are taking any heart or blood pressure
medicines or are pregnant before using.

Hawthorn is a hardy plant and a popular hedgerow tree here in Northern Ireland. Growing up we had a hedge of hawthorn surrounding our cottage, but I had no idea that beyond the fierce thorns was a plant associated with the heart and that its leaves, flowers and berries are all edible and medicinal.

Hawthorn is a plant cloaked in folklore. It was thought to guard the gateway to the faery kingdom and as a result was considered a sacred tree by many. In the spring, it was common to nibble the fresh green buds and leaves for a dose of nutrients and so hawthorn earned the nickname of 'bread and cheese'. While it tastes of neither, the leaves do have a pleasant nutty flavour and the berries are great infused into brandy for a warming, winter heart tonic.

IDENTIFICATION

The hawthorn tree has lobed, green leaves. The flowers are white, often tinged with pink. The small, red berries arrive in autumn.

USES

Hawthorn is an incredible cardiovascular plant. It can help to balance blood pressure, improve circulation and strengthen capillaries and it also helps to promote general heart health. The knock-on effect of a happy heart and cardiovascular system can be felt throughout the body, making hawthorn a powerful plant ally to get to know.

Hawthorn is also a good choice for reducing anxiety and any stress-related palpitations. This is because it contains antioxidant-rich OPCs (oligomeric procyanidins) and essential inflammation-reducing flavonoids, which work on relaxing the nervous system.

Energetically, hawthorn can be an excellent choice when dealing with grief. Try pairing it with rose and oat straw to make a loving and supportive tea during challenging times.

Hawthorn's properties are found in the flowers, leaves and berries, which span across spring, summer and autumn. In spring, harvest the young leaves for salads, and the flowers for tinctures and tonics. Come autumn, the berries are wonderful in infusions, tinctures and hedgerow ketchup – just mind the pips!

HARVESTING & PREPARATION

Ideally, choose a warm, dry morning to harvest. Harvest the flowers in late spring by plucking them off the tree in clusters. Do the same with the leaves and, come autumn, harvest the berries individually from the branches, avoiding any sharp thorns! Dry on trays in a warm, airy place inside or use a food dehydrator set at about 40°C (104°F). Make sure the blossom, leaves and berries are completely dry before storing in airtight glass jars.

Hot Hawthorn Toddy

This deliciously spiced, warming tonic is perfect for the winter months. Here heart-protective hawthorn combines with seasonal spices for a celebratory hedgerow elixir. I love a splosh of this in a cup of hot water with a little honey stirred in. Cheers!

YOU WILL NEED

Freshly picked or dried hawthorn berries
1 cinnamon stick
1 teaspoon finely chopped ginger root
4 whole cloves
1 slice of fresh orange peel
1 slice of fresh lemon peel
Raw honey (preferably local)
Brandy
Clean, dry, wide-mouthed jar with lid
Natural baking parchment
Labels
Muslin (cheesecloth) and fine-mesh strainer
Storage bottle with lid

METHOD

In autumn, when hawthorn berries are ripe, fill the jar three-quarters full with fresh berries (or, alternatively, fill the jar half-full with dried berries).

Add the cinnamon stick, ginger, cloves and orange and lemon peels. Fill the jar one-third full with honey and then pour over enough brandy to cover all the herbs. Stir really well to combine.

Place a square of baking parchment over the mouth of the jar, seal with the lid and label.

Allow to infuse for 4–8 weeks, then strain into a jug (pitcher). If you are using dried berries, you can leave the brandy to infuse for up to 6 months.

You may notice the infusion turning jelly-like during the infusion time. This is due to the pectin in the berries. I find that a quick stir and a dash more brandy loosens it up.

Strain the toddy into a jug to remove the berries and spices. Then funnel into a clean, dry bottle and label.

TO USE

Create a herbal take on a hot toddy by adding 1 tablespoon to a small cup of warm water along with a slice of lemon.

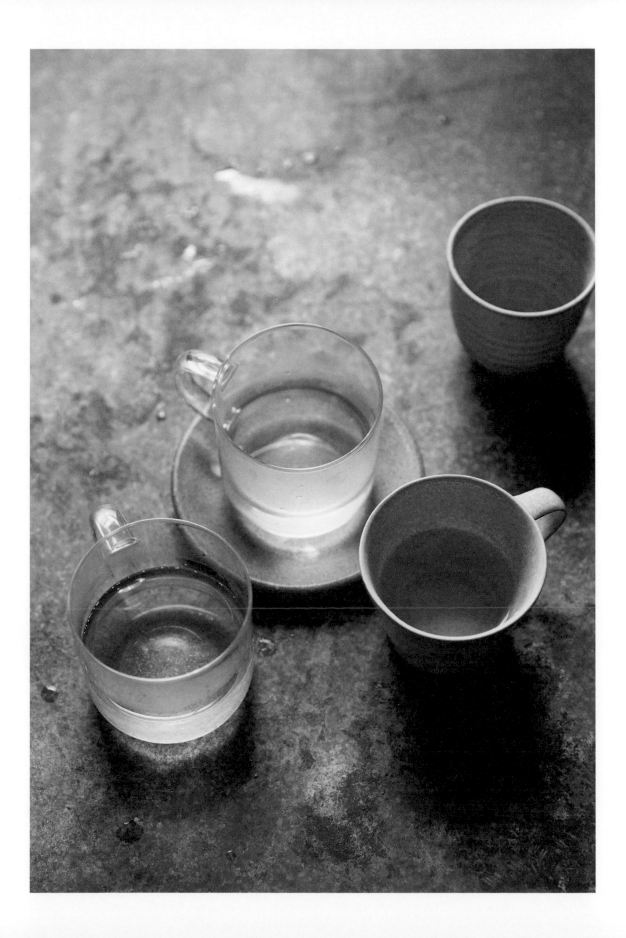

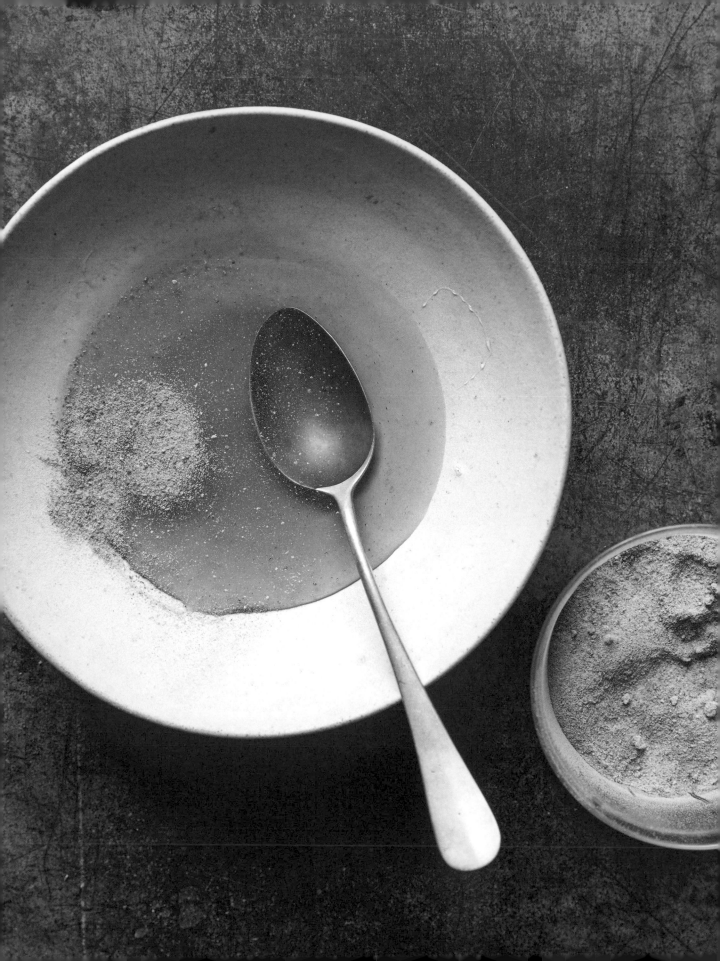

Hawthorn Berry Vinegar

This vinegar, with its ruby-red colour, is the perfect recipe for autumn. If you like to take apple cider vinegar in water daily, substitute it for this healthy alternative. Otherwise, use in any recipe that calls for vinegar.

YOU WILL NEED

Fresh or dried hawthorn berries
Apple cider vinegar (containing the mother)
Clean, dry, wide-mouthed jar with lid
Natural baking parchment
Labels
Muslin (cheesecloth) and fine-mesh strainer
Storage bottle with lids

METHOD

Fill the jar three-quarters full with fresh hawthorn berries, or half-fill it if you are using dried berries. Pour over the vinegar to fill the jar.

Place a square of baking parchment over the mouth of the jar and then screw on the lid (this stops the vinegar from corroding the lid). Label the jar and store for 4 weeks, remembering to shake occasionally.

After 4 weeks, strain the vinegar into a jug (pitcher) using a strainer lined with a piece of muslin to remove the hawthorn berries.

Discard the berries, rebottle the infused liquid and label the jar. Use within 12 months.

Hawthorn Berry Honey

Herbal honeys are such a treat and are a tasty way of consuming herbs daily. This aromatic honey is delicious drizzled over granola or a steaming bowl of porridge, providing not only flavour but also beneficial properties for a healthy heart. If you are making this with store-bought powdered hawthorn berry, you might find the texture a little gritty but not unpleasant. If you want to make your own powder, collect hawthorn berries when they are in season, remove all the pips and dry. Then blitz up in a coffee blender until fine and powdery.

YOU WILL NEED

220 g (7¾ oz) honey
2 tablespoons powdered hawthorn berries
½ teaspoon ground cinnamon or ½ cinnamon stick
Clean, dry, wide-mouthed jar with lid
Label

METHOD

Combine all the ingredients together in the jar and mix well. Seal with the lid and label.

Ideally, let the honey infuse for a couple of weeks before using, although I can never wait and always sneak a taste sooner!

Make sure you give the honey a stir before using, as the powdered herbs tend to accumulate at the top of the jar.

The honey will keep for over a year or longer.

Galium aparine

Cleavers

FAMILY: Rubiaceae

PARTS USED: Aerial parts

ENERGETICS: Cooling and drying

ACTIONS: Anti-inflammatory,
astringent, lymphatic, alterative,
diuretic and tonic

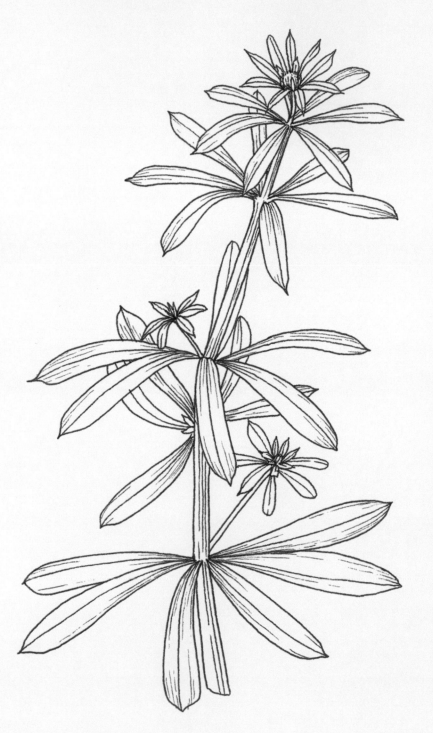

In early springtime, even though the hedgerows look as though they are still deep in slumber, there's life emerging. The little green shoots of cleavers raise their heads above the soil and start the climb upwards towards the strengthening spring sun. I like to fill my foraging basket with handfuls of these shoots during our morning walks. After a long winter my body craves the cleansing properties of cleavers and I like to turn my spring harvest of this herb into a daily infusion, massage oil and a tincture to keep in the store cupboard.

Cleavers is a tremendous spring herb. It emerges from the hedgerows and appears in neglected areas of the garden when little else dares. Bright green and coated in sticky hairs, it's hard to mistake cleavers for any other plant. It has a handful of common names, such as stickyweed and stickybud, all indicating how determined this plant is to cling on to everything it touches. Unchecked, cleavers will wind its way through vegetation, using its tiny hooks to clamber up. Luckily, this tenacious weed is easy to pull up and also has some interesting uses in the herbalist's kitchen!

IDENTIFICATION

Cleavers has hollow, square-shaped stems. The whole plant is coated in little hooked spines that cling to other plants, helping it to grow upwards. The leaves are narrow and grow up the stems in circular whorls. Each whorl has 6–8 leaves. The flowers of cleavers are tiny and white. Later in the season, cleavers produce small, round, green fruits that are bi-lobed. These are also covered in tiny hooks.

USES

A timely lymphatic herb, cleavers is the perfect plant for early spring when our bodies can feel sluggish after a long winter, and we might find ourselves dealing with puffiness, dry patches and dull skin. Acting as a kind of herbal spring cleaner for our systems, it helps eliminate waste and toxins from the body and gives our lymphatic system a good boost, which in turn boosts immunity. Traditionally, cleavers has been used to reduce swollen lymph nodes and to treat tonsillitis. With its diuretic action, it is also potentially a good herb to use to help ease urinary tract conditions.

A lovely ritual for spring is to use a cleavers-infused oil before a bath or shower. Rub the herbal-infused oil in using brisk, circular motions over the entire body, working from the feet upwards and towards the heart. Rinse off with warm water. The combination of the cleavers and the massage helps circulation, skin health, immunity and to combat water retention.

With its silica content and lymphatic action cleavers is also a great herb for chronic skin issues such as acne, psoriasis and eczema. If you struggle with these, try drinking the Cleavers Springtime Infusion (see page 80) daily, taking a cleavers tincture or using the Spring Greens Vinegar on page 165.

HARVESTING & PREPARATION

My favourite time to harvest cleavers is in early spring when the growth is still lovely and young, and it is perfect for using fresh. Later in the season, as the cleavers begins to flower, you can harvest this herb and dry it for tincturing. Once cleavers has gone to seed, it is past its best. However, the seeds can be picked and dry-roasted to make a tasty, although slightly time-consuming, substitute for coffee.

Cleavers Springtime Infusion

Once you start seeing the new spring growth of cleavers, make sure you grab a big bunch to make this cleansing infusion. It's refreshing and delicious to drink daily and will help give your system a gentle boost ready for a busy season ahead!

YOU WILL NEED

Fresh cleavers
Water
Fresh lemon
Fine-mesh strainer

METHOD

Gather a handful of young cleavers – make sure there are no roots! Give the cleavers a quick wash and then chop them roughly.

Put the chopped cleavers in a glass jar or jug (pitcher) and fill with water. Cover and leave for an hour, then place in the fridge overnight.

Strain the infusion into your mug to remove the cleavers. Then, serve with a squeeze of lemon.

TO USE

Try drinking up to three glasses of this infusion daily throughout spring.

Skin Support Tincture

This skin-loving tincture will help support the liver and lymphatic system as well as aid detoxification and cleansing. This is my favourite tincture for early spring when my body feels in need of a good spring clean. If you would rather avoid alcohol, you can infuse the herbs in this recipe in vinegar instead for a similar result.

YOU WILL NEED

1 part dried cleavers – aerial parts
1 part dried chickweed – aerial parts
½ part dried calendula flowers
½ part dried dandelion root
Strong vodka (at least 40% alcohol)
Clean, dry, wide-mouthed jar with lid
Natural baking parchment
Labels
Muslin (cheesecloth) and fine-mesh strainer
Storage bottle with a lid

METHOD

Half-fill the jar with all the herbs, then pour over the vodka until the plant material is completely covered.

Place a square of baking parchment over the jar and seal with the lid. Label and leave to infuse for 4 weeks.

Once the infusion time is over, pass the tincture through a strainer lined with a piece of muslin to remove the herbs. Use a funnel to transfer the strained tincture into a bottle, then label and date.

TO USE

Take 1 teaspoon up to three times a day when needed. Consult a GP before using if you have any liver, kidney or gallbladder issues. Caution required if pregnant or nursing.

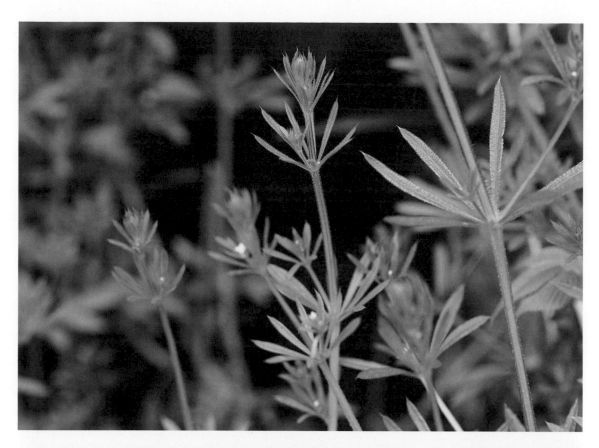
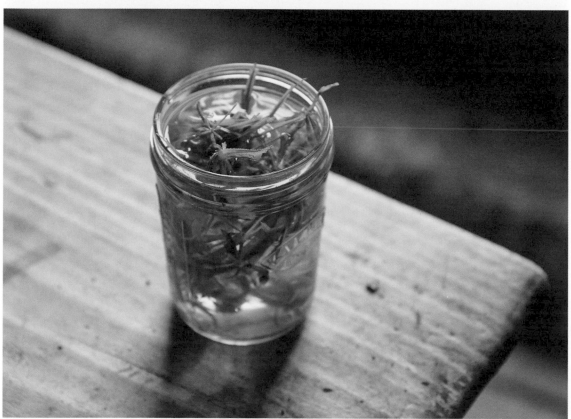

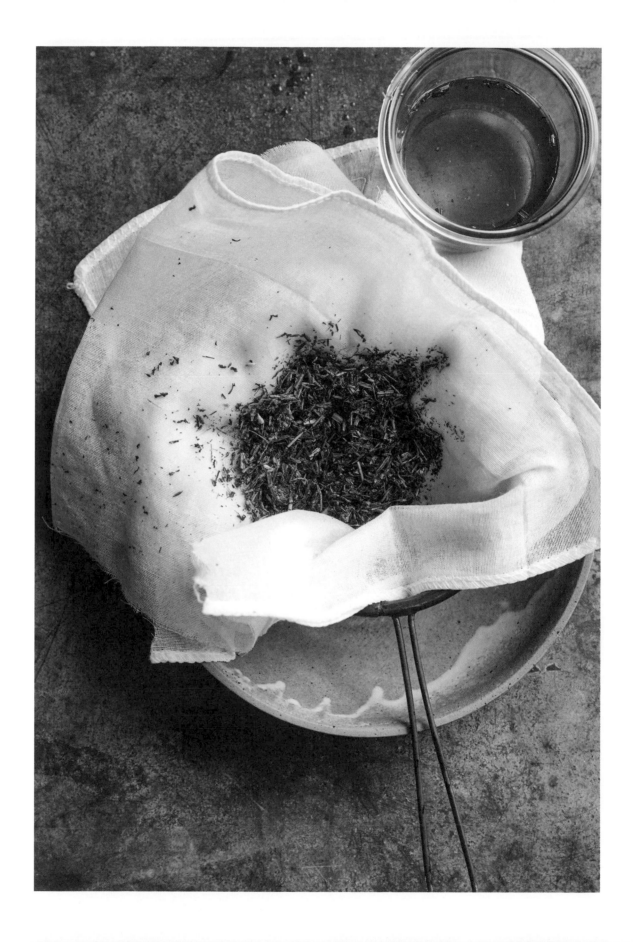

Invigorating Cleavers Massage Oil

Cleavers make an ideal oil for self-massage during the winter and spring. Its lymphatic and astringent effects help rid the body of retained water and promote healthy skin. The addition of essential oils gives this massage oil a beautiful, uplifting fragrance and additional invigorating benefits.

YOU WILL NEED

For the infused cleavers oil:

Your choice of carrier oil, such as sunflower oil
Dried cleavers
Wide-mouthed jar with lid
Muslin (cheesecloth) and fine-mesh strainer
Storage bottle with lid
Label

For the massage oil:

5 drops juniper berry essential oil
6 drops lavender essential oil
4 drops ginger essential oil
Storage bottle with lid
Label

METHOD

Half-fill the wide-mouthed jar (ensuring it is clean and dry first) with dried cleavers. Pour over the carrier oil (in this case, sunflower oil) to fill the jar. Make sure all the herbs are completely covered in oil. Seal with the lid and label.

Allow the oil to infuse in a cupboard for 4–6 weeks, giving it a little shake every few days or so.

When the infused oil is ready, pass through a strainer lined with a piece of muslin into a jug (pitcher). Squeeze the muslin tightly to ensure all the oil has been removed from the cleavers.

Use a funnel to transfer the infused oil to a clean, dry bottle, seal and label with the contents and date.

TO MAKE THE MASSAGE OIL

Pour 3 tablespoons of the infused cleavers oil into a clean, dry bottle. Add the juniper berry, lavender and ginger essential oils to further encourage circulation and to boost the detoxifying effect of the massage oil.

TO USE

Rub a small amount of the massage oil between your palms. Apply in a circular motion over the entire body (avoiding the face) either before or after a shower or bath.

If you are pregnant or nursing, omit the essential oils.

Lavandula angustifolia

Lavender

FAMILY: Lamiaceae

PARTS USED: Flowers

ENERGETICS: Warming

ACTIONS: Antispasmodic, antimicrobial, carminative, emmenagogue, hypotensive and nervine

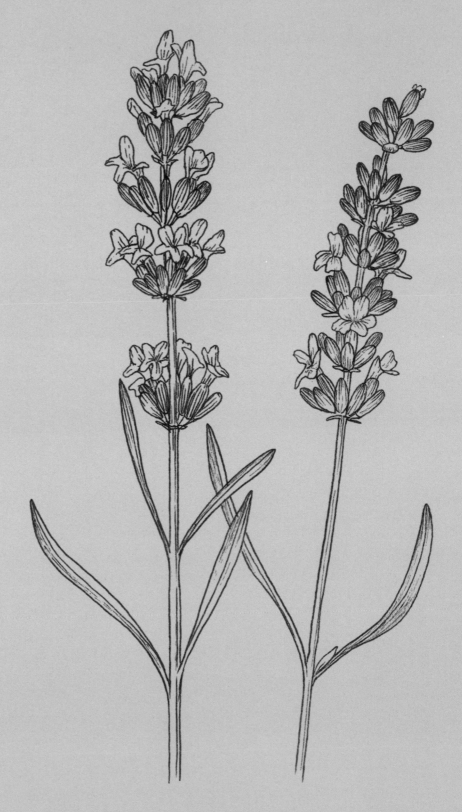

The beautifully scented lavender is a true workhorse herb. Not only does it look wonderful in a garden border, but it also has plenty of uses in a home apothecary and in the kitchen. Its name is derived from the Latin 'to wash', suggesting its longstanding affinity with cleansing.

Lavender plays a huge role in my home. In summer, it is harvested and dried in bundles. The dried flowers are placed in small linen pouches which are then tucked under our pillows at night to help with sleep. I also use powdered lavender as an ingredient to gently exfoliate my skin. Lavender essential oil is always taken with me in case of cuts, scrapes and bites. Lavender even sneaks its way into puddings and cakes, scenting everything it touches with that nostalgic fragrance that's so evocative of a hot summer's day.

IDENTIFICATION

Lavandula angustifolia is a perennial herb that's popular in warm, sunny gardens. It has long, greenish-grey stems topped with lavender-hued flowers which appear in a whorl pattern.

USES

Lavender's antimicrobial, calming and pain-relieving qualities make it a superb herb for minor burns, cuts, scrapes and insect bites. In fact, lavender essential oil was used during the Second World War as a treatment for soldier's war wounds. Dilute a drop of good-quality essential oil with some sunflower or olive oil and dab it on any minor cut to promote healthy healing. Even better, make a strong lavender salve that you keep in your first aid kit. I use my All-Purpose Healing Salve (see page 86) for everything from scrapes and stings, and as a temple balm for aiding relaxation. In addition to its wound-healing properties, lavender also has a balancing effect on the skin as well as being antimicrobial. As a result, it's my favourite herb to include in an all-natural DIY deodorant.

Although most people think lavender has a beautiful scent, flies don't! Try keeping bunches around the house, especially in the kitchen in the summer months, to keep them at bay.

Moths also aren't a fan of lavender, so creating herb-filled pillows with catnip and lavender is a great way to repel moths and keep clothes smelling fresh. I love to make these pillows and keep them snuggled into my folded woolly jumpers.

Of course, lavender is renowned for soothing anxiety and calming a busy mind, making it a great bedtime herb, and its gentle touch means it is a good one for children, too. I enjoy using a lavender-infused oil as a post-bath massage oil, or directly in the bath. Otherwise, a lavender hydrosol works wonders as a baby-safe bedroom and pillow spray. A simple lavender tincture or glycerite can be an aid for easing nervous tension-related headaches and helping to induce a good night's sleep.

HARVESTING & PREPARATION

Harvest lavender just before the flowers open. To dry and store lavender, cut long lengths of stem so the herb can be dried in bunches. If you are using a food dehydrator, remove the majority of the stalk and dry the flowers at around 35°C (95°F).

Garden Blossom Glycerite

The blossoms in this glycerite are gentle mood boosters and help calm nervous tension. The alchemy of the garden flowers is sure to bring sunshine back into your day.

YOU WILL NEED

Fresh or dried lavender flowers
Fresh or dried rose petals
Small sprig of mint (preferably flowering)
Vegetable glycerin (food-grade)
Clean, dry, wide-mouthed jar with lid
Labels
Muslin (cheesecloth) and fine-mesh strainer
Amber glass storage bottle with lid

METHOD

Fill the jar three-quarters full with a equal parts fresh lavender flowers and rose petals, or half-fill the jar if using dried flowers. Add a small sprig of mint blossom.

If you are using fresh flowers, pour over enough glycerin to fill the jar, covering all the herbs. If using dried flowers, dilute 3 parts glycerin with 1 part water and fill the jar with this, covering the herbs. Mix well.

Seal the jar with the lid and label. Allow to infuse for 4 weeks, topping up with more glycerin if needed.

Strain the mixture into a jug (pitcher) using a strainer lined with a piece of muslin. Funnel into the bottle, seal with the lid and label.

The glycerite should last 1–2 years.

TO USE

Take ¼–1 teaspoon up to three times a day in water when needed.

All-Purpose Healing Salve

This recipe is a must-have for any gardener and home cook. It works really well at soothing mild rashes, scrapes, bruises and mild burns. The lavender helps to keep the area clean, soothes and also encourages repair.

YOU WILL NEED

1½ teapoons beeswax pellets
3 tablespoons lavender-infused extra-virgin or sunflower oil
   (see page 44 for how to make an infused herbal oil)
7–50 drops lavender essential oil
Double boiler
Salve jar or tin with lid
Label

METHOD

Set up a double boiler over a low heat, then melt the beeswax in the top section (ensuring this is clean and dry first). Pour in the lavender-infused oil and stir to melt together. Once the beeswax has melted, remove the double boiler from the heat.

Stir in a suitable dilution of essential oils (see the Essential Oil Dilution Chart on page 51). I personally like to add 50 drops for an approximate 4% dilution.

Pour the salve mixture into the jar or tin and seal with the lid. Allow to cool and harden for 24 hours before labelling and using. The salve will last at least 12 months.

TO USE

Dab a bit of salve gently on the area. Repeat as needed.

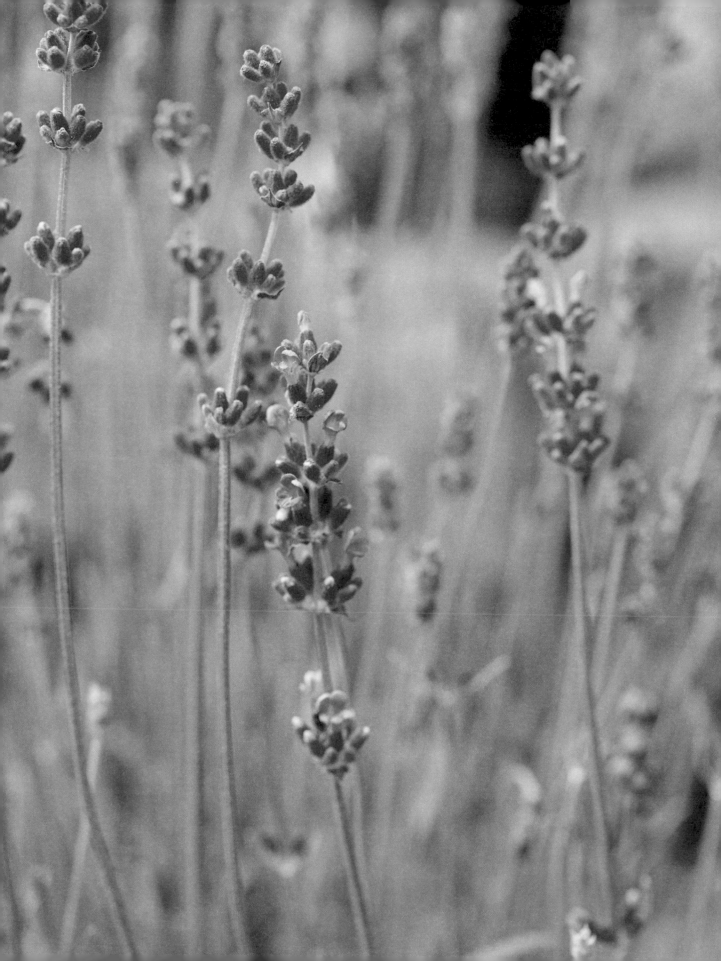

Lavender Deodorant

I love this gentle, natural version of deodorant. You can add whatever essential oils you want, but lavender is ideal for its scent and oil-balancing and antibacterial qualities.

YOU WILL NEED

3 tablespoons lavender-infused coconut oil (see Method)
3 tablespoons shea butter
3 tablespoons bicarbonate of soda (baking soda)
3 tablespoons arrowroot powder
12 drops lavender essential oil
Muslin (cheesecloth) and fine-mesh strainer
Shallow jar or container with lid
Label

METHOD

To make the lavender-infused coconut oil, slowly melt 125 g (4 oz/1 cup) of coconut oil in a small saucepan, add 3 tablespoons of dried lavender flowers and allow to infuse gently over the heat (don't allow to simmer) for around 2 hours.

Strain into a jug (pitcher) using a strainer lined with a piece of muslin. Pour the oil into a jar, seal with the lid and allow to solidify.

For the lavender deodorant, add the shea butter and solidified lavender-infused coconut oil to a bowl and mash with a fork until well combined.

Stir in the bicarbonate of soda and arrowroot powder. Add the lavender essential oil and mix to combine.

Scoop the deodorant into a shallow jar or container with a lid, and then label.

TO USE

Rub a small quantity of the deodorant into the armpits.

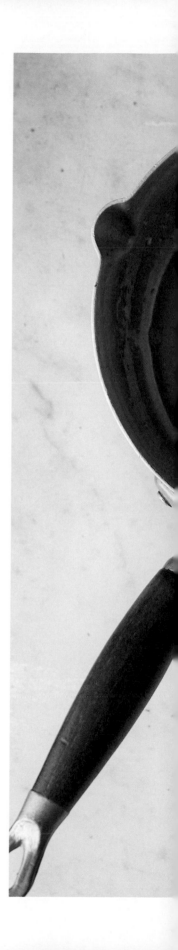

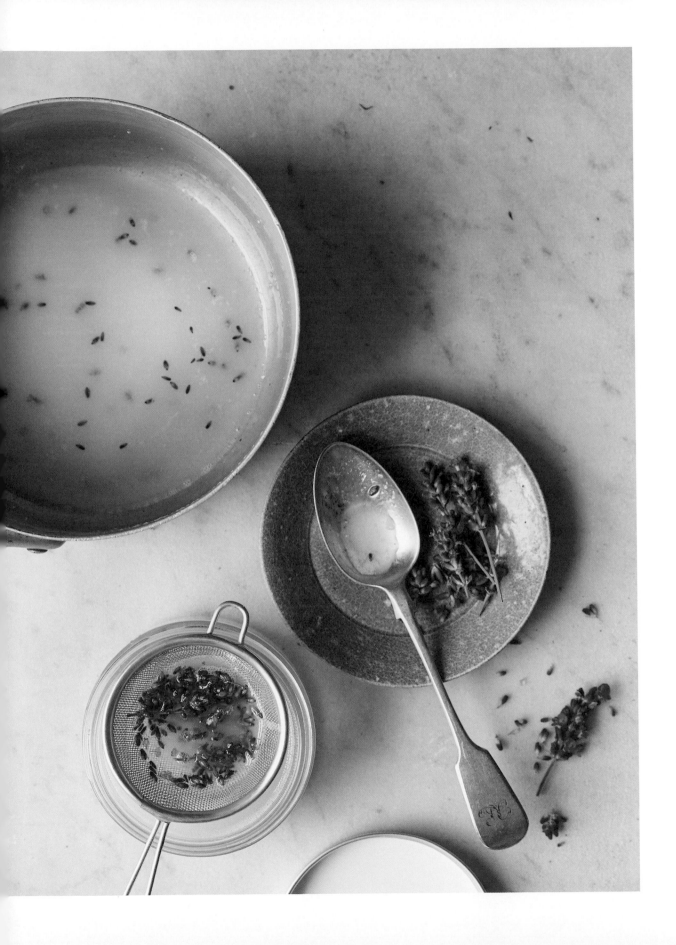

Melissa officinalis

Lemon Balm

FAMILY: Lamiaceae

PARTS USED: Leaves

ENERGETICS: Cooling and drying

ACTIONS: Antimicrobial, antiviral,
antidepressant, carminative, nervine,
diaphoretic and antispasmodic

SAFETY: Avoid use if you have
a hypothyroid condition.

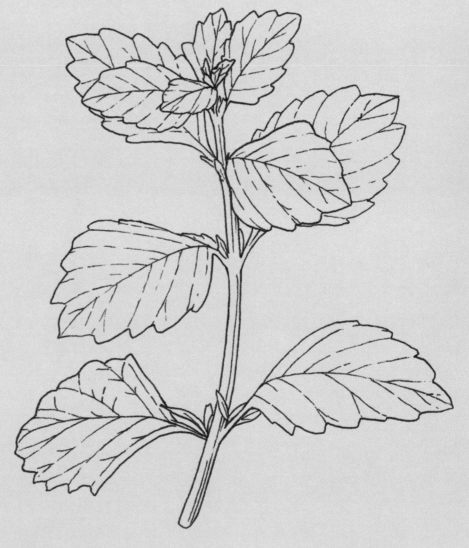

Lemon balm has been in my life for as long as I can remember. My parents always had a huge bush of it growing in our herb bed and I would often be sent out to harvest a bunch. It is similar in appearance to its relative mint, so I wouldn't be sure I had the right herb until I had nestled my face deep into the green bouquet I had just picked. The minute I smelt the fresh lemon scent I knew I had lemon balm. When I had my own garden, the first thing I grew was my own lemon balm plant. It's an easy plant to establish in a garden and its beautiful and strong aromatics make it a wonder in the kitchen and home apothecary.

As a mother, I see lemon balm as an essential part of my home remedies. For my two small boys, lemon balm is a great choice for bedtime, and I recommend every parent learn how to grow and use it.

IDENTIFICATION

Lemon balm looks similar to mint with square stems and slightly furry leaves which are toothed and opposite. This perennial herb looks beautiful in any garden.

USES

Lemon balm is the herb to reach for to soothe nerves, relax overexcited little ones, help ease anxiety and raise the spirits. Its delicious and uplifting lemony taste is a joy to sip and a great choice alongside lemon verbena to drink in the midst of winter, when we can all feel the effects of SAD, or before a big event when nerves and worries can start to get the best of us. As a mild and safe nervine, it's a beautiful herb for anyone who finds nodding off to sleep a struggle or has unsettled nights. Try a lemon balm glycerite before bedtime to help promote a deep and restful sleep or try adding a bundle of the fresh herb to a night-time bath and soaking in the wonderful aroma.

Lemon balm is also known as a gentle antispasmodic and a good herb to calm a nervous tummy or bouts of colic. Due to its volatile oils, bitters and astringent tannins, lemon balm can really help to ease the symptoms of irritable bowel syndrome in a gentle and effective way by acting on not only the digestive system but also on the mind and nerves. Try drinking a delicious lemon balm tea combined with chamomile to stop those nervous butterflies and palpatations or mild tummy rumbles (see my Tummy Calm Tea on page 93).

Another use for lemon balm is to calm viral skin issues such as cold sores. A simple lemon balm infused oil in a lip balm should help calm and clear the skin.

HARVESTING & PREPARATION

Harvest lemon balm before it begins to flower. Dry the leaves in bunches upside down somewhere dry and airy or, alternatively, dry in a food dehydrator set at 38°C (100°F) overnight or until the herb is completely dry and crisp to the touch – but make sure the leaves are still very fragrant. Store in a dry, airtight jar and use within a year. Note that lemon balm is at its most potent when fresh, so make sure you try making a fresh lemon balm glycerite and a tea from the just-picked leaves.

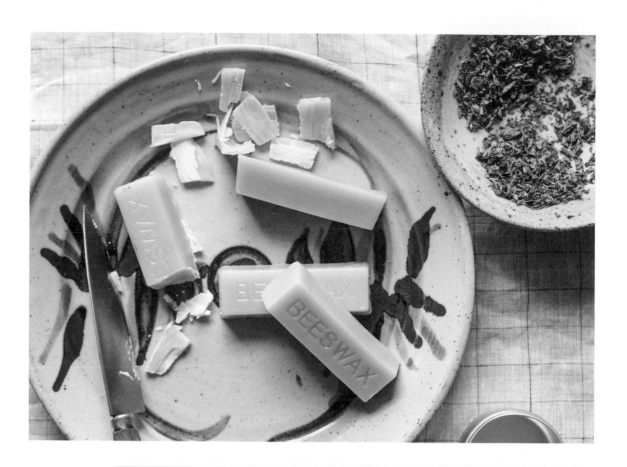

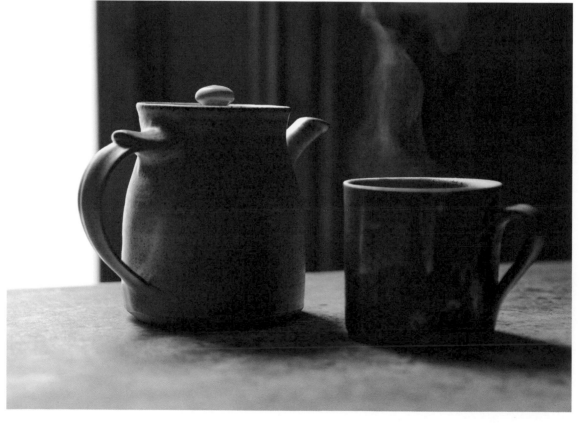

Lemon Balm for the Lips

Lemon balm has antiviral actions, which makes it a great choice for healing uncomfortable cold sores or dry, flaking lips. Thanks to the lemon balm and essential oil, this lip balm is perfect for healing any skin irritations. The waxes and oils also act as a protective, moisturising barrier for the lips or any dry patches of skin. If you want to use this balm on children, omit the essential oil.

YOU WILL NEED

1 teaspoon beeswax
2 teaspoons lemon balm-infused sunflower oil
   (see page 44 for how to make an infused herbal oil)
1 teapoon shea butter
3 drops *Eucalyptus radiata* essential oil
Double boiler
1 x 15 ml (½ oz) lip balm tin
Labels

METHOD

Melt the beeswax in a double boiler over a low heat. Once the wax has almost melted, add the lemon balm-infused sunflower oil and shea butter and stir until all the wax has melted. Stir in the *Eucalyptus radiata* essential oil.

Remove the double boiler from the heat and carefully pour the fragrant liquid into the tin.

Seal the tin with the lid and allow the balm to set for around 2 hours before labelling and using.

Tummy Calm Tea

If you suffer from a nervous tummy or stress-related IBS (irritable bowel syndrome), then lemon balm could become a favourite herb of yours. Its calming and antispasmodic effects when used alongside chamomile are wonderful at soothing an uncomfortable, gassy tummy. This tea is also lovely for calming the mind before bed and is safe for children to use, too.

YOU WILL NEED

1 teaspoon dried chamomile flowers
2 teaspoons dried lemon balm leaves
Boiling water
Raw honey, preferably local (optional)
Tea strainer

METHOD

Add the herbs to a tea strainer set in a mug (or to a teapot if you want to make a larger quantity).

Pour boiling water over the herbs and allow to infuse for 10 minutes.

Remove the herbs and enjoy the tea. Stir in a little honey if desired.

If using fresh herbs, double the quantity of herbs.

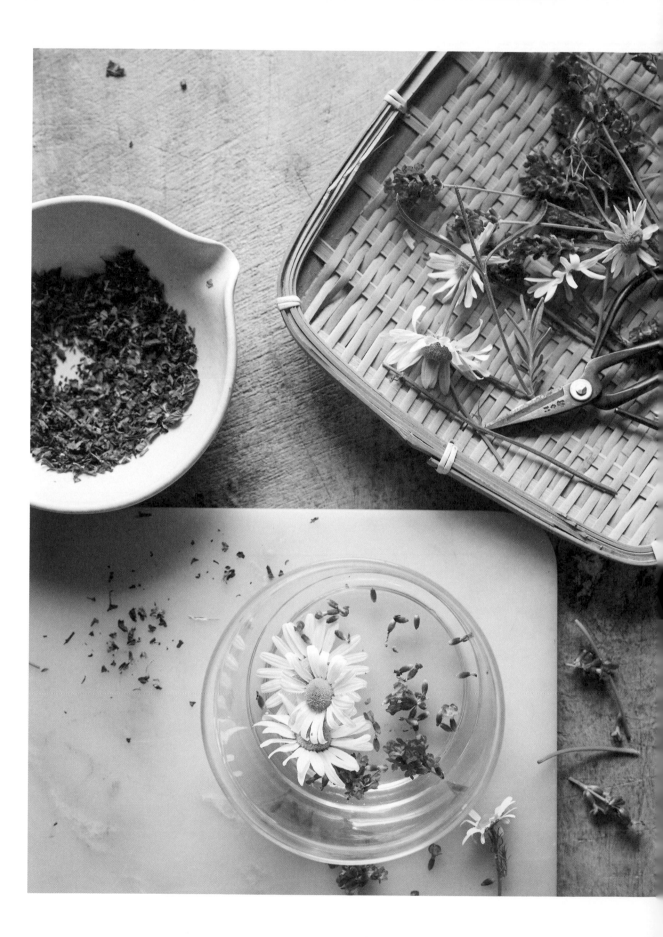

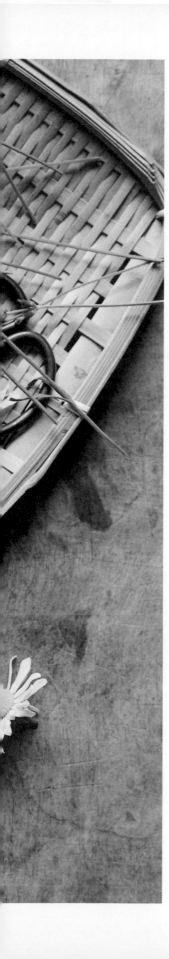

Night-time Glycerite

This sweet-tasting glycerite will help lull even the busiest of minds into a gentle sleep. A glycerite is a tincture made with glycerin as opposed to alcohol and is what I reach for with children, especially as it also has a sweeter flavour.

YOU WILL NEED

1 part fresh or dried lemon balm leaves
½ part fresh or dried chamomile flowers
½ part fresh or dried lavender flowers
Vegetable glycerin (food-grade)
Clean, dry, wide-mouthed jar with lid
Labels
Muslin (cheesecloth) and fine-mesh strainer
Amber glass dropper bottle

METHOD

Fill the jar three-quarters full with fresh lemon balm, chamomile and lavender. If you are using dry herbs, half-fill the jar.

Pour over enough glycerin to fill the jar completely. If you are using dried herbs, dilute 3 parts glycerin with 1 part water and pour this over the herbs to fill the jar.

Stir well to release any air bubbles, then seal with the lid and label. Allow to infuse for 4 weeks, topping up with more glycerin if necessary.

Strain the glycerite into a jug (pitcher) using a strainer lined with a piece of muslin. Funnel into the dropper bottle and label. The glycerite should last 1–2 years.

TO USE

For adults, take ½–1 teaspoon up to three times a day in water when required. For children, consult a clinical herbalist for exact dosage depending on weight and age.

Mentha piperita

Peppermint

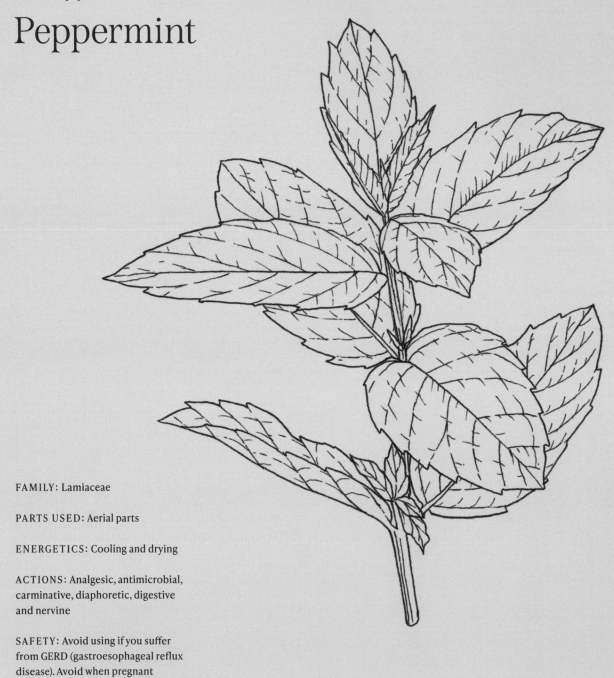

FAMILY: Lamiaceae

PARTS USED: Aerial parts

ENERGETICS: Cooling and drying

ACTIONS: Analgesic, antimicrobial, carminative, diaphoretic, digestive and nervine

SAFETY: Avoid using if you suffer from GERD (gastroesophageal reflux disease). Avoid when pregnant or nursing. Not for young children.

Chocolate, apple, spearmint, basil ... I think I might have a bit of an obsession with collecting different varieties of mint. I keep them in a cluster of terracotta pots (mint will take over a garden bed, so a container is always a good idea) outside my red cottage door. If I had to choose one variety for use in a home apothecary, I would choose peppermint (*Mentha piperita)*. This mint is strong and has a classic, clean and fresh minty taste and aroma that works well in many recipes.

I use mint in a variety of ways: ground up into a powder as an ingredient in a natural toothpaste, for an after-dinner tea or as part of an invigorating body scrub. Its cooling effect makes it a wonderful summer companion and it has the added benefit of clearing the mind and helping with focus – I often diffuse peppermint essential oil with lemon in the summer months while I work on my podcast.

Of course, mint is also a delicious culinary herb. It tastes amazing muddled into cocktails and mocktails and simply diced finely and mixed with a good-quality vinegar as a fresh sauce alongside any kind of roast.

IDENTIFICATION

Peppermint has a square stem and simple, opposite, dark green leaves with jagged edges. When crushed the herb releases an unmistakable and powerful mint scent. In summer it has purple flowers.

USES

Mint is famed for its affinity with the digestive system. Just think of those hard mint sweets given out in restaurants or peppermint capsules used as a popular treatment for IBS (irritable bowel syndrome). Mint has a relaxing effect on the digestive system. It stimulates the digestion and improves absorption. Mint contains menthol and other volatile oils which can help to relieve nausea. Peppermint is an excellent choice in cases of excess gas, gastric spasms and discomfort. It works well as a strong tea for this, so keep a jar of dried peppermint for use whenever you've over-indulged.

Mint is also clearing to the sinuses and airways, helping to provide relief from nasal congestion, while its antimicrobial action makes it a good herb for treating infections and colds settling in the upper respiratory system. In this case, you could add some bunches of peppermint leaf, along with fresh rosemary and thyme, to some hot water in a bowl and, using a towel to cover your head, bend over and inhale the steam. This is a great way of opening up the airways and delivering the beneficial qualities of the herbs to the sinuses.

I also turn to mint when I feel a thumping headache coming on. As an anodyne or pain reliever it can bring some respite from the discomfort while the cooling and opening qualities of peppermint really help to ease overall tension and bring some much-needed relief. A minty balm rubbed onto the pulse points and shoulders is one of my favourite ways of using mint for this.

HARVESTING & PREPARATION

Mint is a prolific herb, growing abundantly throughout the warmer months. Harvest peppermint before it flowers and dry it in bundles. As with other herbs it can also be dried in a food dehydrator set at about 37°C (99°F). Dried mint still contains plenty of potent benefits and will last at least a year in an airtight jar.

Iced Morning Infusion for Sluggish Starts

If you've woken up on the wrong side of bed, try this uplifting, joyful tea blend to help clear your head, focus the mind and bring energy to the body. A fantastic alternative to coffee, this infusion has a refreshing citrus flavour and slightly earthy, bitter element due to the rosemary, which satisfies my coffee cravings. While you can drink this warm in the cooler seasons, it tastes delicious as an iced tea, too.

YOU WILL NEED

1 teaspoon dried peppermint leaves
1 teaspoon dried lemon verbena or lemon balm leaves
Small pinch dried rosemary leaves
Boiling water
Tea strainer

METHOD

Add the peppermint leaves, lemon verbena or lemon balm leaves, and rosemary leaves to a tea strainer set inside a small teapot or mug.

Pour boiling water over the herbs and allow to infuse for 10 minutes.

Remove the herbs and enjoy the infusion warm.

Variation

To make an iced herbal tea, allow the infusion to cool for a few minutes, then pour over a cup of ice cubes. Squeeze in some fresh lemon juice and stir in 1 teaspoon of honey for sweetness. In summer, you can make your tea with freshly harvested leaves.

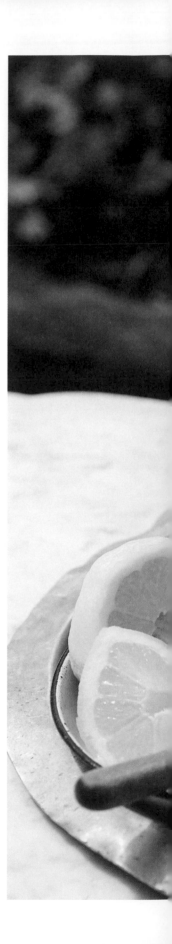

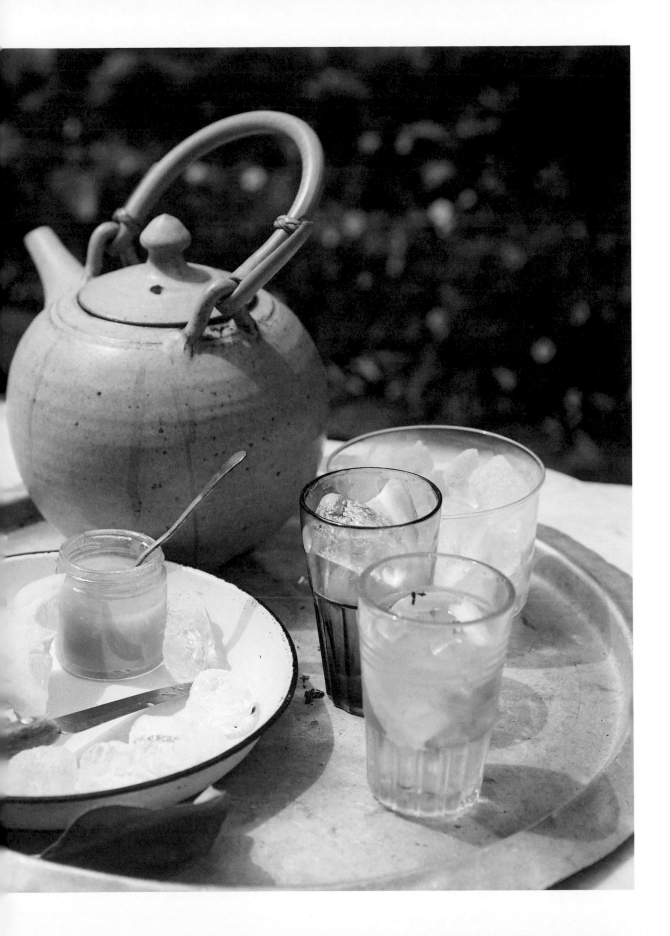

Tension Relief Balm

All kinds of tension-related aches and pains, such as headaches and neck tension, will be soothed by this plant-packed balm. To use, just rub a small amount over the back of the neck or onto the temples or pulse points. For menstrual cramps, top with a warm heat pack for extra relief. This balm is not suitable for children or for those pregnant or nursing.

YOU WILL NEED

1 tablespoon beeswax pellets
3 tablespoons infused herbal oil, using sunflower oil infused
   with equal parts dried mint leaves, yarrow leaves and flowers,
   and lavender (see page 44 for how to make an infused
   herbal oil)
85 g (3 oz) shea butter
30 drops peppermint essential oil
35 drops lavender essential oil
Small container(s) with lid
Label

METHOD

Melt the beeswax in a double boiler. Once the wax has melted, add the infused herbal oil and shea butter. Once everything has melted, remove from the heat.

Add the essential oils and mix to combine. Pour the balm into your choice of container(s).

Allow the balm to cool and harden for 24 hours before labelling and using. This balm should last for 12 months.

Hair Booster Tonic

If you suffer from a dry, itchy scalp or dull, brittle hair, give this hair tonic a go! It is packed full of aromatic herbs that help balance the scalp and tone and strengthen the hair. This vinegar hair tonic helps seal the hair shaft, giving shine to the hair. Rosemary and thyme are said to improve circulation, which can encourage hair growth.

YOU WILL NEED

Dried nettle leaves
Dried rosemary leaves (use chamomile flowers for blonde hair)
Dried thyme
Dried peppermint leaves
Apple cider vinegar
Spray bottle

METHOD

First make a herbal vinegar from apple cider vinegar infused with equal parts of nettle, rosemary, thyme and peppermint, following the instructions on page 37. Infuse the vinegar for 4 weeks.

When you want to wash your hair, pour 60 ml (2 fl oz/¼ cup) of the herbal vinegar into a spray bottle, then top with 250 ml (12 fl oz/1 cup) of water.

After shampooing your hair, pour or spray the vinegar over your clean hair and massage into the roots.

Rinse the vinegar out with cool water. Dry and style your hair as usual. Repeat weekly.

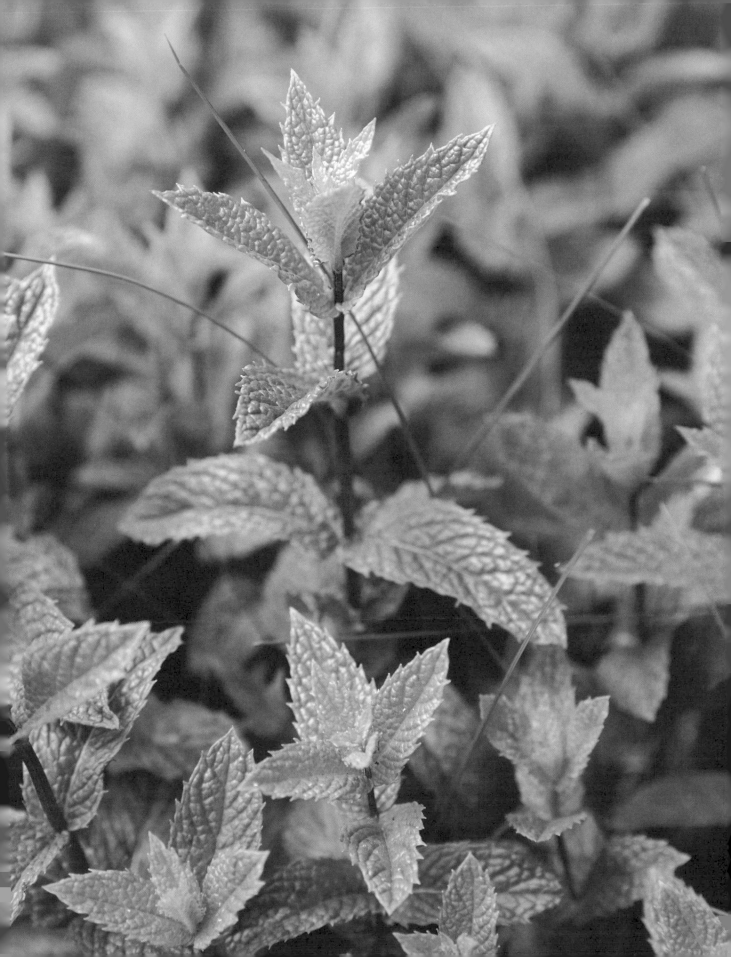

Pinus spp.

Pine

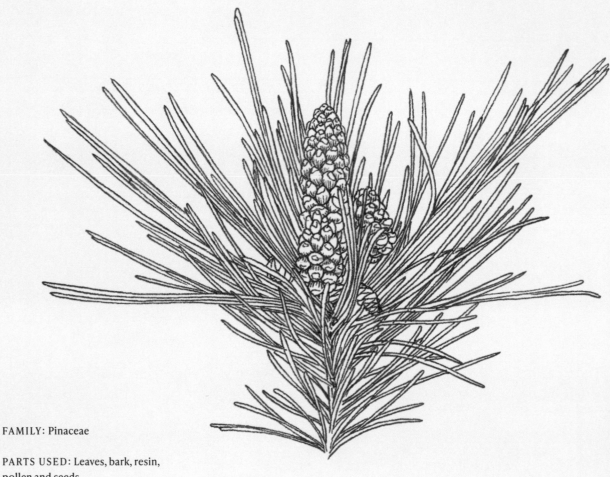

FAMILY: Pinaceae

PARTS USED: Leaves, bark, resin, pollen and seeds

ENERGETICS: Drying and warming

ACTIONS: Antimicrobial, nutritive, expectorant and vulnerary

SAFETY: Do not use pine when pregnant and use with caution while breastfeeding. Do not mistake pine for yew, as yew is fatally toxic.

The pine tree, with its majestic stance and spiky needles, might not be the first garden edible that springs to mind. However, pine trees have many healing properties and, of course, the most incredible aromatics that make me think of log cabins, roaring fires and winter celebrations.

Prized in the Nordic countries for its high vitamin C content, pine is traditionally used in teas, ales and, of course, the pine nuts (from the *Pinus pinea*) are used in pesto. Even the bark, resin and pollen are all edible. What an amazing plant!

IDENTIFICATION

The pine is a large tree, conical in shape. It has orange flowers in late spring and early summer, which develop into green cones that eventually harden up and turn brown. *Pinus sylvestris* has grey-green needles set in pairs (some other species of *Pinus* may have up to five needles in a bundle) attached directly to the stem in a paper-like sheath.

USES

Pine, with its clearing scent, can be an ideal plant to reach for if you have a cough, cold or congestion. Pine has an expectorant quality which can help thin and shift unpleasant mucus from the lungs. One of my favourite ways to take pine is by brewing up a strong cup of pine needle tea combined with a spoon of delicious honey. Team this with a pine-infused chest rub and you should feel relief in no time at all and smell like a winter forest.

Apart from its affinity with the respiratory system, pine is also good at reducing inflammation of the skin. Its antimicrobial, pain-reducing and vulnerary actions make it a great choice for any healing salve. While you can make a salve with an infused pine oil and beeswax, you could also look at using pine resin. Resin is a bit like a tree's version of a plaster. It seals wounds on the bark and the antimicrobial qualities stop bacteria and infection occurring. With sympathetic harvesting we can use resin for the same things. I particularly like to use a resin-based salve when healing wounds left over from nasty splinters, to warm up cold aching joints in winter, speed up the healing of stubborn old cuts to calm irritated skin.

HARVESTING & PREPARATION

Pine can be harvested all year round. In spring and summer, the needles have a lighter flavour, but it is said that there is more vitamin C in the needles in the winter. The resin can also be harvested throughout the year, but be wary of damaging the tree or overharvesting. Ideally, harvest resin that has already dripped down the bark. You can remove this with a knife and store it in a jar. Dry needles on a tray in a warm, airy room or in a food dehydrator, set at 38°C (100°F)

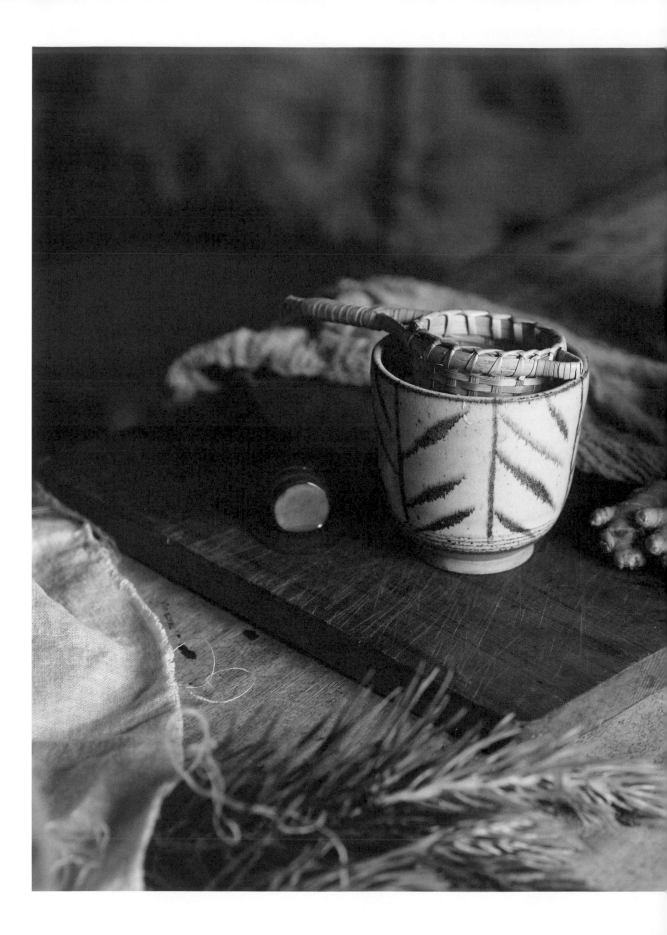

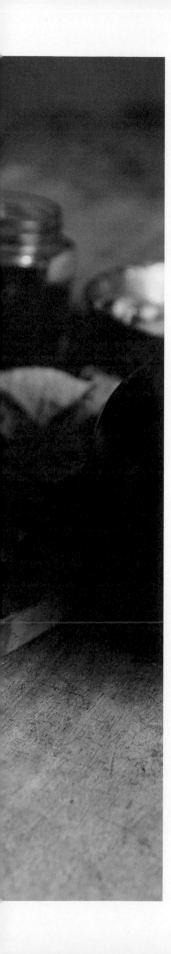

Pine & Ginger Winter Tea

This simple, aromatic tea is a beautiful and medicinal brew that is well matched to the winter season. The strong, clearing aroma of pine helps to open the airways and support a healthy respiratory system while the ginger heats the body.

YOU WILL NEED

2–3 teaspoons chopped freshly picked pine needles
2.5 cm (1 in) piece of fresh ginger root, chopped into small pieces
Boiling water
1 teaspoon raw honey
Tea strainer

METHOD

Place the pine needles and ginger in a tea strainer set in a mug and pour over some just-boiled water. Put a small saucer over the top of the mug to trap in the amazing aromatics of the pine.

Allow to infuse for 10 minutes, then remove the strainer, stir in the honey, inhale and enjoy!

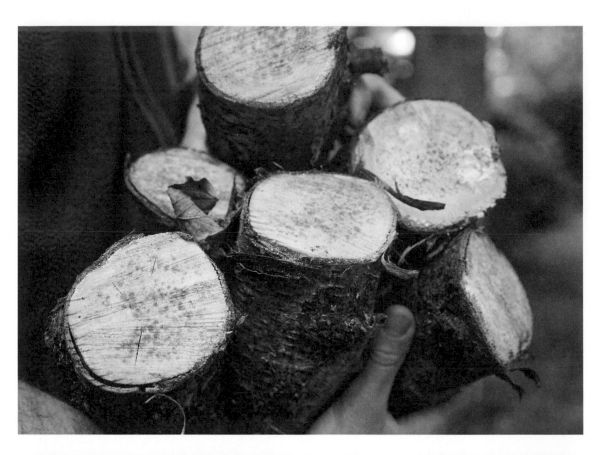
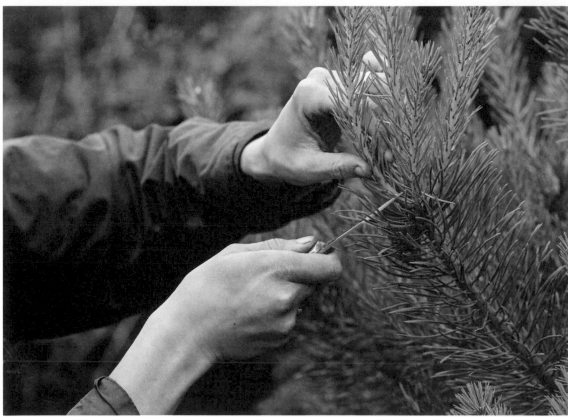

Forest Skin Oil

Wake up your mind and body with a full-body rub down using this invigorating and refreshing skin oil. Perfect to use pre-shower, just rub a tablespoon over the skin in circular motions to boost the lymphatic system and open the airways.

YOU WILL NEED

Freshly harvested pine needles
Carrier oil, such as sunflower or olive oil
Clean, dry, wide-mouthed jar with lid
Muslin (cheesecloth) and fine-mesh strainer
Storage bottle with lid
Labels

METHOD

Finely chop the pine needles, then add to the jar until it is about three-quarters full.

Pour over the carrier oil and stir with a clean chopstick. Add more oil if necessary, making sure all the needles are covered. Seal the jar with the lid and label.

Leave to infuse in a warm place for up to 4 weeks. During this time all the aromatics and benefits from the pine needles will seep into the carrier oil.

Once the 4 weeks are over, strain the mixture into a jug (pitcher) using a strainer lined with a piece of muslin. Funnel the oil into a bottle, seal with the lid and label. Discard the pine needles or add to the compost bin.

TO USE

Pour a small amount of oil into your palm and warm between your hands. Rub in circular motions from your feet upwards to boost circulation. You can use this oil before or after a shower or bath.

Woodsman's Pine Tree Salve

Thanks to pine's vulnerary and antimicrobial effects, this salve works well on eczema, psoriasis and any itchy, dry skin. I love keeping a small tin of this in my pocket to keep chaps and wounds at bay – especially in winter when your hands are dry and any cuts or splinters seem slow to heal.

YOU WILL NEED

30 ml (1 fl oz/½ cup) Forest Skin Oil (see left)
60 ml (2 fl oz/¼ cup) pine resin
28 g (1 oz) beeswax pellets
15 drops sweet orange essential oil
10 drops spruce or pine essential oil
Double boiler
Muslin (cheesecloth) and fine-mesh strainer
Salve tins or jars with lids
Labels

METHOD

Add the forest skin oil and pine resin to a double boiler. Bring to a gentle heat and melt the resin. Use an old spoon to stir, as the resin may stick to the spoon.

Once the oil and resin have melted together, if you've used home-foraged resin, pour the mixture into a jug (pitcher) through a strainer lined with a piece of muslin to remove any bark. If you've used store-bought resin, this step is not necessary.

Return the oil and resin mix to the double boiler and add the beeswax, allowing it to melt. Remove from the heat.

Add the sweet orange and spruce or pine essential oils and stir.

Pour into the tins or jars and seal. Allow the salve to cool and harden for 24 hours before labelling and using.

The salve will last for at least 12 months.

Plantago major or
Plantago lanceolata

Plantain

FAMILY: Plantaginaceae

PARTS USED: Leaves and seeds

ENERGETICS: Cooling and moistening

ACTIONS: Antimicrobial, astringent,
anti-inflammatory, demulcent, diuretic,
expectorant, nutritive and vulnerary

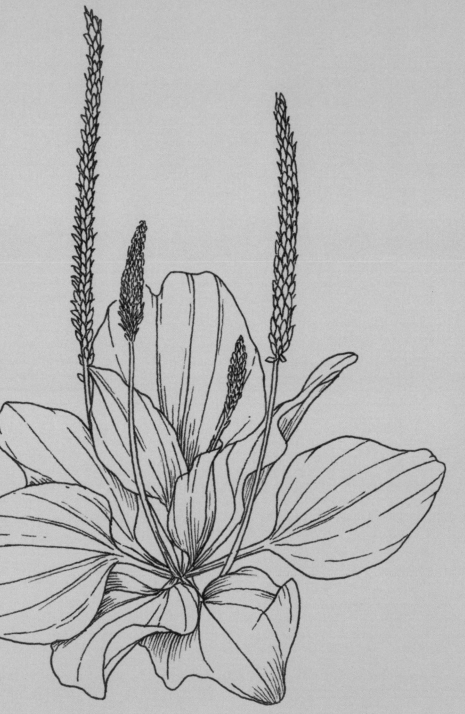

Despite its humble appearance, I've always had a soft spot for plantain. Its peculiar looking flower heads have intrigued me since childhood, and they were often used as a makeshift plaything in games. Plantain is the kind of weed that I adore and one all gardeners should definitely learn to love and use. While it's easy to overlook and doesn't add much visual appeal to a garden, it is also prolific and easy to find, usually near paths or places that get a bit of wear and tear.

Most importantly, behind its plain appearance is a dependable healing herb. I'm often grabbing leaves of plantain to help remove stuck thorns and splinters and to soothe and heal stings. Its gentle soothing action also makes it a nice addition to a healing skin oil.

IDENTIFICATION

Plantain has green leaves with very distinct parallel veining, which gives the leaf a ribbed appearance. *Plantago lanceolata* has narrow leaves and tall, leafless stalks with narrow, oval flower heads. *Plantago major* has broad leaves. Always check with a good plant guide when identifying a herb for the first time. A selection of excellent guides is listed in the Resources section at the back of the book.

USES

Plantain really comes into its own as a first aid plant. It's effective at drawing out thorns, splinters and stings and can be used to heal the area in question quickly. With its antimicrobial and astringent qualities, plantain works effectively to draw out the object and helps to heal the wound, too.

My favourite way to use plantain is by making a DIY poultice on the go. Thorns, bites, scratches, stings ... these all usually happen when I'm out gardening or when the children are playing outside. Plantain to the rescue! I grab a couple of the leaves, pop them into my mouth and chew them up. While this may seem counterintuitive, it actually creates a lovely poultice. It also creates a substance called aucubigenin which is very antibacterial. Once the plantain has broken down a bit, I spit it out and use this 'spit poultice' to cover the wounded area. Often, I'll use a fresh plantain leaf to seal this on top. The poultice works at drawing out the thorn and preventing infection. I urge you to try it next time you get a splinter or thorn stuck in a finger! If the thought of creating a spit poultice leaves you feeling a bit queasy, then you can make a version from the dried leaves (see page 110).

Plantain is also a gentle astringent and expectorant and its soothing qualities make it a good herb to reach for when you have a mild cough or cold. For relief, try drinking plantain leaf as an infusion, one cup up to three times a day, or make up a batch of my Mullein & Plantain Cough Syrup (see page 169).

HARVESTING & PREPARATION

Harvest leaves without overhandling them, as they have a tendency to bruise. Spread them out on a tray to dry in a warm, airy room or, alternatively, dry them in a food dehydrator set at 43°C (109°F).

Drawing Poultice for Stings & Splinters

I seem to get splinters and various scrapes and cuts on my hands almost constantly. I think it's part of the joys of farm and garden life! So, learning how to use plantain to clean the area and draw out any pesky thorns is a handy skill to master. This recipe has two parts. First of all, you make a salted plantain wound rinse. This will help clean the area well. The second part involves making a soothing poultice that helps to heal the area further and will aid the removal of any stings or splinters.

YOU WILL NEED

For the wound rinse:

6–8 fresh plantain leaves or 1 heaped tablespoon dried plaintain
Boiling water
1 teaspoon salt
Fine-mesh strainer

For the poultice:

1 tablespoon fresh or dried plaintain
Warm water
Pestle and mortar

METHOD

Part 1: Making the wound rinse

Make a plantain infusion by chopping the leaves well and adding them to a cup of just-boiled water (reserve a tablespoon of the freshly chopped plantain leaves).

Alternatively, use dried plantain instead of fresh plantain leaves.

Allow the plantain to infuse for 20 minutes, then strain into a jug (pitcher) and compost the plantain.

Stir in the salt. Once the mixture is cool enough, soak a cloth in the plantain and salt water and use to clean the area gently.

Part 2: Making the poultice

Add the fresh or dried plantain to a mortar. Add enough warm water and use the pestle to create a rough paste.

Now place the finely chopped plantain paste over the wound and wrap in place with a clean bandage or cloth.

Leave the poultice on for at least 10 minutes. You can repeat the poultice as often as needed.

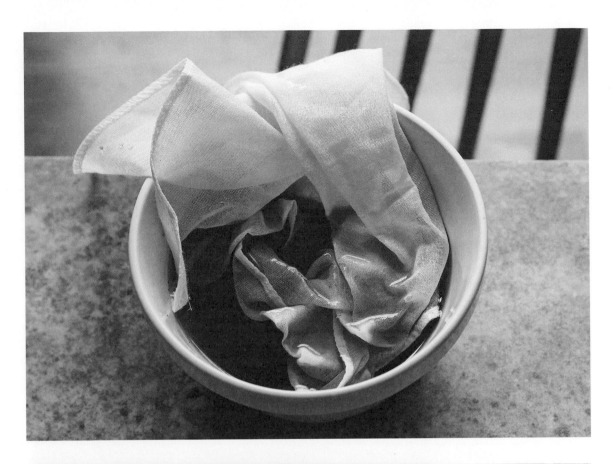

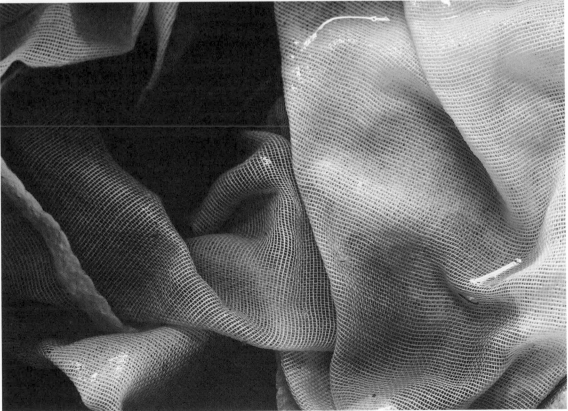

Plantain & Daisy
Bruise Salve

This simple salve is the one to reach for when you have bumps, bruises, grazed knees, splinters, bites and rashes. It's soothing, healing and antimicrobial. Daisy is a great local (and more sustainable) alternative to arnica and is said to help heal bruises. I find it works a treat on any bruises that my rambunctious toddler gets!

YOU WILL NEED

3 tablespoons herbal-infused oil, using sunflower or olive oil
    infused with equal parts dried plantain leaves and daisy
    flowers (see page 44 for how to make an infused herbal oil)
1½ teapoons beeswax
7–15 drops lavender essential oil
Double boiler
Salve jar or tin with lid
Label

METHOD

Melt the beeswax in a double boiler over a low heat. Once the beeswax starts to melt, add the infused herbal oil. Let the wax and oil melt together, stirring if necessary.

Once the wax and oil have melted together, remove from the heat and add the lavender essential oil. Stir to combine.

Pour the finished salve into the jar or tin and seal with the lid. Allow the salve to cool and set for 24 hours before labelling and using.

The salve will last up to a year.

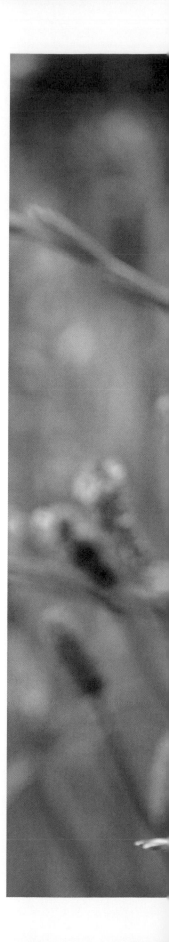

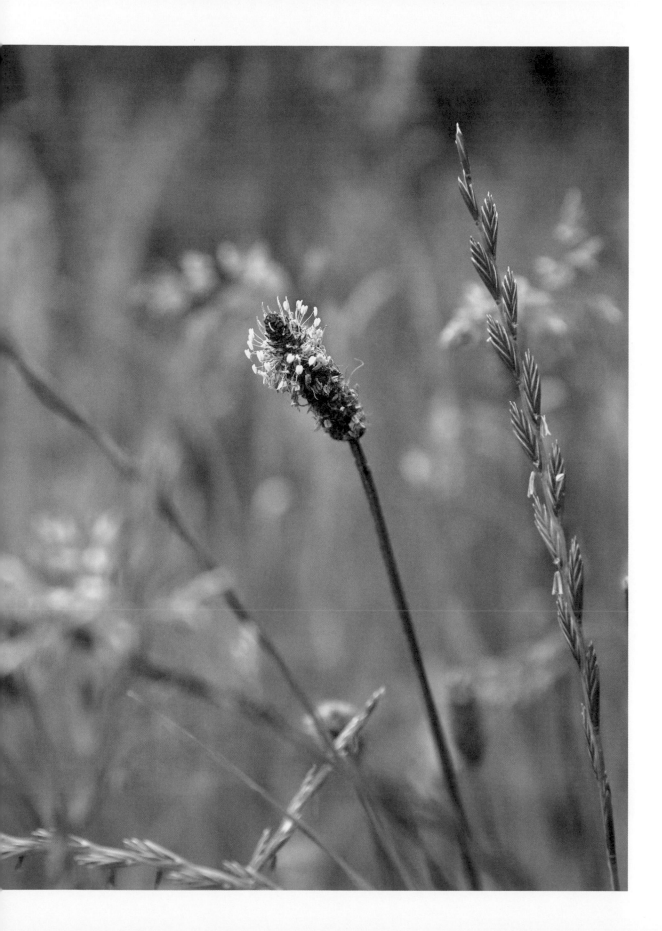

Rosa spp.

Rose

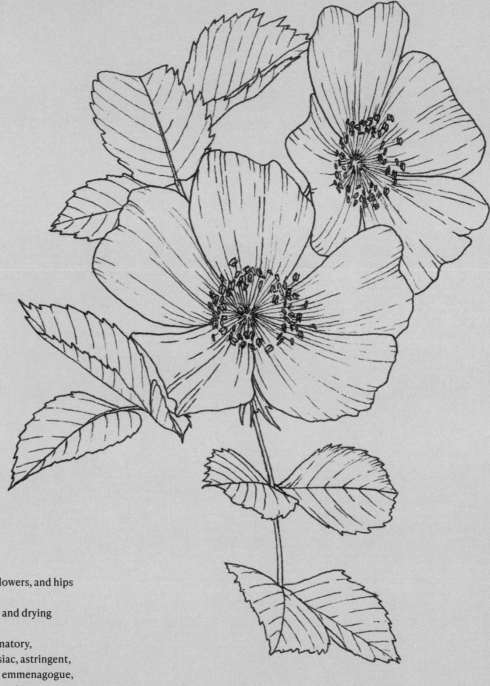

FAMILY: Rosaceae

PARTS USED: Leaves, flowers, and hips

ENERGETICS: Cooling and drying

ACTIONS: Anti-inflammatory, antispasmodic, aphrodisiac, astringent, cardiovascular, diuretic, emmenagogue, hypotensive, tonic and nervine

SAFETY: Avoid large doses if pregnant.

There is something so exquisite about the rose with its velvety soft petals and intoxicating fragrance. Traditionally associated with Aphrodite, the goddess of love, the rose symbolises passion, desire, love and sexuality within many cultures. However as a medicinal plant the rose has multiple uses and both its petals and its fruit are a mainstay in my home apothecary.

In the *Rosa* genus you'll find wild and cultivated varieties. The dog rose (*Rosa canina*) or *R. rugosa* can be incorporated into hedgerows for a visually appealing and fragrant effect. We have many wild roses, alongside the rambling honeysuckle, planted into ours here on the farm.

Cultivated roses, the ones with multiple petals and grown with much care in our gardens, are also edible, but my favourite will always be the hardier wild varieties.

IDENTIFICATION

Roses have many curved thorns running up their stems. The pretty blooms appear in early summer, with wild roses having five petals that are usually pink and sometimes white. In autumn, wild roses carry oval fruits called hips which are orangey red in colour and contain hairy seeds. Their leaves are toothed and arranged on alternate sides of the stem. Make sure your garden roses haven't been sprayed if you plan on using them for remedies and in the kitchen.

USES

The herbal actions of the rose are pretty impressive. It's nutrient-rich, astringent, diuretic and anti-inflammatory and also used for uplifting the spirits, for grief, PMS, upset tummy, sore throats, colds and during the menopause. Roses can be used in tinctures, glycerites, teas, honeys, oxymels, syrups, vinegars and hydrosols, as a flower remedy and an essential oil.

Rose hips are commonly known as being a good source of vitamin C. During the Second World War, rosehip syrup was given to children to ensure they were consuming ample vitamin C, as imported fruit was harder to come by. Children were encouraged to collect rose hips for the Ministry of Health. In 1941, there were 200 tonnes of hips collected and processed into a National Rose Hip Syrup which was available at chemists for families to purchase as a supplement.

The leaves of the rose are full of tannins which makes it a good alternative to black tea, having a similarly astringent effect but without the caffeine. It is also a good tea to take to soothe an upset tummy.

From an energetic perspective rose is like a warm, motherly embrace – it is soothing, heart-opening, softening and gentle. Rose is full of femininity, comfort and tenderness. It can be used to help heal a broken heart, to find calm after trauma and emotional upheaval, give love and self-care, and provide us with a feeling of warm comfort.

HARVESTING & PREPARATION

The best time to harvest rose petals is mid-summer. Collect the petals on a dry morning. Gently pull off the petals, leaving behind the calyx of the rose. Dry on a tray in a warm, airy room or at a low heat (about 34°C/93°F) in a food dehydrator. When harvesting rose hips wait until the hip is completely ripe, usually in autumn, and bright orange or red. Remove the seeds and irritating hairs from the hip before use. The hips can also be dried as above but use a slightly higher heat (43°C/109°F) in the dehydrator.

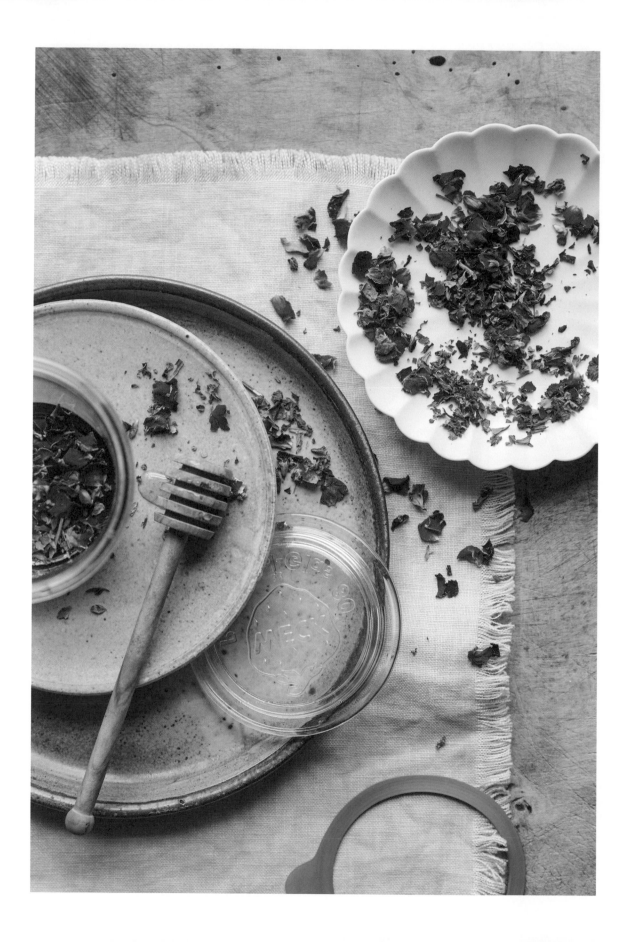

Rose & Lemon Balm Honey

Herbal honeys are among my favourite concoctions, especially when rose is included. There is something almost magical about spooning the golden, viscous syrup into a cup of steaming water, or pouring it in ribbons over a milky pudding. It's so soothing, fragrant and calming, and it's also incredibly easy to make. With the addition of relaxing lemon balm this honey is pure heaven!

YOU WILL NEED

Dried rose petals (crushed into small pieces)
Dried lemon balm leaves (crushed into small pieces)
Raw runny honey
Clean, dry, wide-mouthed jar with lid
Label
Fine-mesh strainer (optional)

METHOD

To make rose honey, half-fill the jar with rose petals and lemon balm leaves. Pour over the honey. Stir with a spoon or chopstick to ensure the petals are all coated and to remove some of the air bubbles. Add extra honey, if needed, ensuring all the petals are covered.

Seal the jar with the lid, label and leave to infuse for 4–6 weeks and then the honey is ready to be eaten.

You can leave the herbs in the honey if you wish or alternatively warm the honey slightly and strain through a fine sieve.

The herbal honey will last at least a year.

Nourish Tea

This tea is fragrant, uplifting and nourishing. Oat straw acts as a tonic, chamomile soothes frayed nerves, rose adds its loving energetics, while verbena or lemon balm add further relaxing properties as well relaxing the body. This tea is perfect to drink before bedtime or whenever you need a gentle, restorative pick-me-up.

YOU WILL NEED

1 part dried chamomile flowers
1 part dried oat straw
½ part dried rose petals
½ part lemon verbena or lemon balm leaves
Boiling water
Clean, dry jar with airtight lid
Tea strainer

METHOD

Mix the herbs together in the jar, ensuring you use an airtight lid.

Put 2 teaspoons of the herb mix in a tea strainer set in a mug and pour over boiling water.

Leave to infuse for 10 minutes, then remove the herbs.

TO USE

Drink up to three cups a day.

Rose Hip Syrup

When autumn creeps in and the hips of the rose bushes become bright and fat, it's time to make this delicious syrup packed with vitamin C and essential antioxidants.

YOU WILL NEED

125 g (4 oz) freshly picked or dried rose hips
500 ml (16 fl oz/2 cups) water
62–125 g (2–4 oz/½–1 cup unrefined caster (superfine) sugar,
    maple syrup or honey
1 tablespoon brandy, vodka or herbal tincture (optional)
Muslin (cheesecloth) and fine-mesh strainer
Syrup bottle with lid
Label

METHOD

Add the rose hips and water to a saucepan. Bring to a boil, then simmer for 20 minutes until the rose hips have softened and the water is reduced by half.

Strain the rose hips into a jug (pitcher) using a strainer lined with a piece of muslin.

Measure out 250 ml (8½ fl oz/1 cup of the herbal liquid and return to the saucepan. Add the sweetener. If using sugar, return the pan to the heat until the crystals have dissolved.

Remove from the heat, add the alcohol and stir well.

Funnel the syrup into the bottle, seal with the lid and label.
Use within 4 weeks

TO USE

Take 1 tablespoon a day to help ward off colds and flus.

I like to make this using Hawthorn Berry Honey (see page 77). It gives a delicious flavour and has additional benefits.

Rose Hydrosol

There is nothing quite like a homemade rose hydrosol. Freshly made hydrosol can be diluted at a ratio of 1:10 as an incredibly aromatic tea or used as a facial toner to tighten and protect the skin.

YOU WILL NEED

Fresh rose petals, clean and unsprayed
Ice cubes
Clean brick or sturdy heatproof ramekin
Large saucepan with lid
Heatproof bowl that fits inside the saucepan
Turkey baster
Storage bottle with lid
Label

METHOD

Place the brick or heatproof ramekin in the base of the large saucepan. Add the rose petals and cover with water up to the level of the brick/ramekin.

Place a bowl on top of the the brick/ramekin, making sure it's heatproof. Invert the saucepan lid and place cubes of ice in the lid indentation.

Slowly bring the pan to a simmer. As the water heats the plant material, condensation will appear on the pan lid and slowly drip into the bowl, collecting aromatic floral water.

When the lid begins to fill up with melted ice, remove with a turkey baster and replace with fresh ice cubes.

Once the bowl has collected enough rose hydrosol, remove the pan from the heat, carefully funnel into a clean, dry storage bottle and label. Store the hydrosol in the fridge for up to 2 weeks.

This process will take about an hour and you will have to replace the ice a few times through this time.

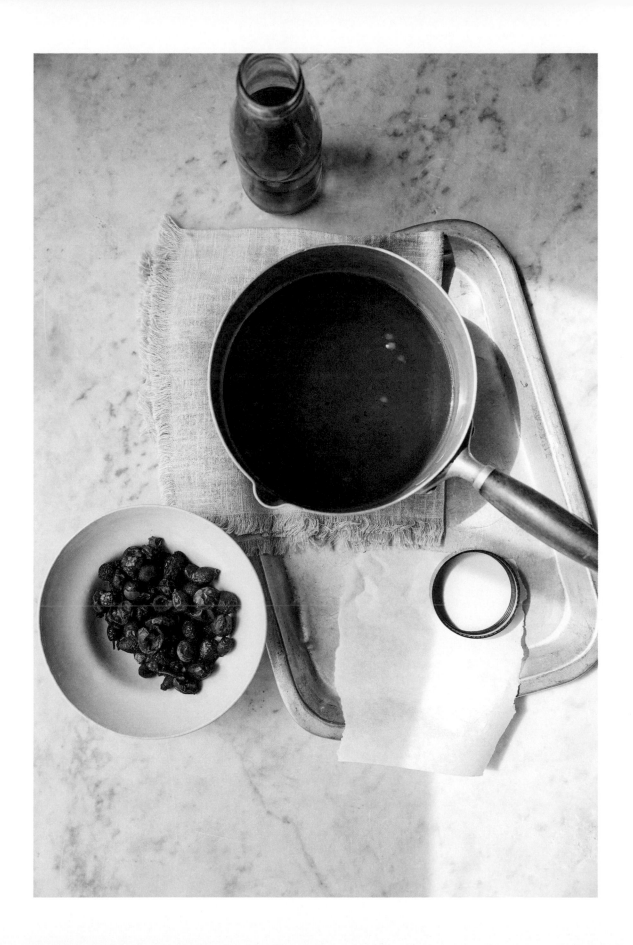

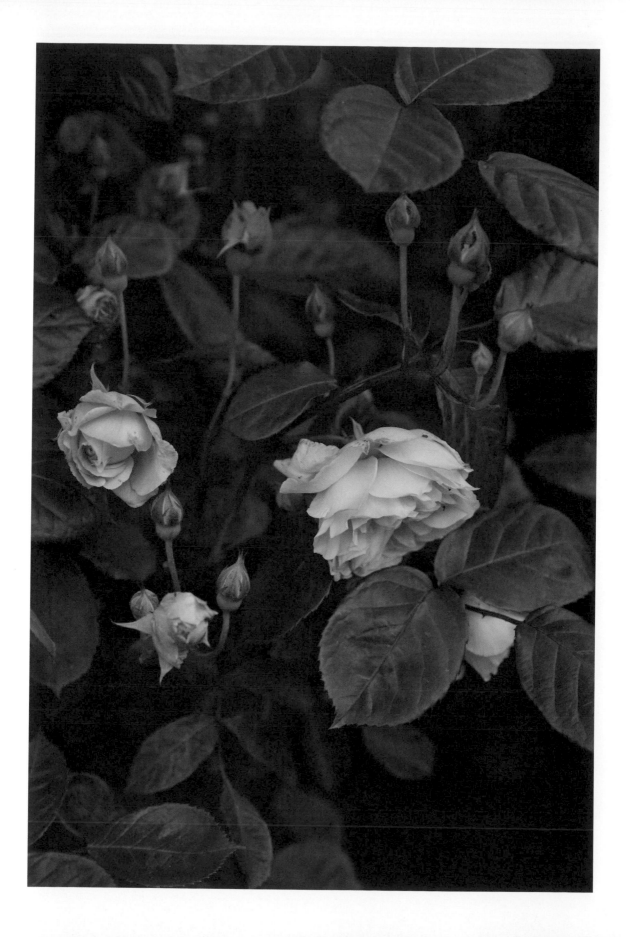

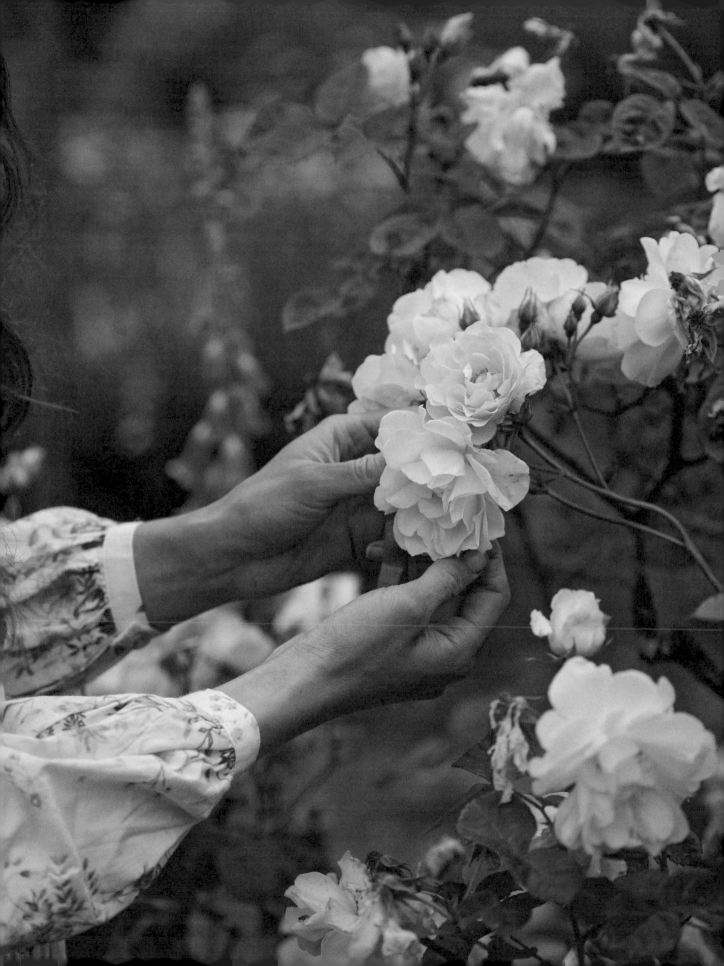

Rosmarinus officinalis

Rosemary

FAMILY: Lamiaceae

PARTS USED: Leaf

ENERGETICS: Warming and drying

ACTIONS: Anti-inflammatory, antimicrobial, antioxidant, antispasmodic, antidepressant, brain tonic, carminative, circulatory stimulant, decongestant, digestive, emmenagogue, hepatic, nervine and rubefacient

SAFETY: Avoid using larger or medicinal quantities during pregnancy and lactation.

Even just a passing whiff of rosemary takes me straight to the Mediterranean from where it originates. Its botanical name means 'dew of the sea', a hint that rosemary thrives especially well in warm, sunny coastal spots. Full of aromatic oils, rosemary finds its way into my kitchen daily. In summer, when it's at its most abundant, big bunches are harvested and hung up to dry. In the colder seasons, dried stems are plunged into bottles of golden rapeseed oil along with a curl of lemon peel and given as gifts. Personally, I find a cup of hot rosemary tea is just the ticket for a stuffy nose and fuggy head, or for when I need to focus my mind.

IDENTIFICATION

This woody perennial shrub grows well in areas of full sun. It has needle-like leaves that sit opposite each other on the stem. Rosemary flowers in mid-summer and these purple blooms are tasty and edible in salads.

USES

With its spiky needles and strong aromatics, rosemary is unmistakable. Not only is rosemary delicious used in cooking, but it also has uses as an antimicrobial, memory booster, hair tonic and circulatory stimulant, making it a wonderful herb to grow in your garden. Rosemary's famous nickname is the 'herb of remembrance', suggesting it has a particular affinity with focus and memory. Said to enhance the cellular uptake of oxygen, rosemary can help with headaches and keeping focus sharp. It is the perfect herb to inhale when you're working long hours at a desk and need to keep your mind on the job. Try a potent cup of rosemary tea or, alternatively, inhale rosemary essential oil to utilise its benefits next time a deadline is looming.

Rosemary is also an excellent digestive herb. Its astringent and antimicrobial effects aid overall gut health, and it also encourages a healthy digestive system while relieving gas and bloating. It is often recommended in cases of headaches brought on by indigestion. It also has liver-protective qualities and is very high in antioxidants.

There are a couple of herbs renowned as hair tonics and rosemary is one of them. Said to help with hair loss and general scalp health, as well as helping to subtly darken hair, a simple rosemary oil can be massaged into the scalp weekly and washed off with a gentle shampoo. Try my Hair Booster Tonic on page 100, which is made with nettle as well as rosemary for even more benefits.

HARVESTING & PREPARATION

Harvest by cutting the long stems, tying them up in bunches and hanging them somewhere warm, dry and airy to dry out. Alternatively, dry the needles on a tray in a warm, airy room or in a food dehydrator set at 35°C/94°F.

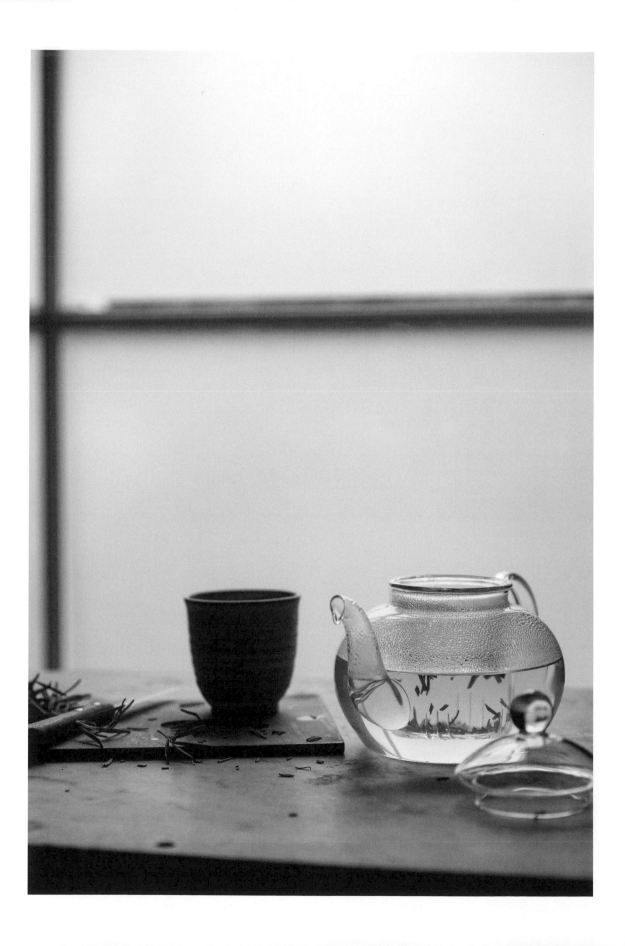

Quick Remedy for Stuffy Sinuses

If you're feeling bunged up, this tea will certainly give some relief. Rosemary's decongestant actions help shift some of the congestion. Make sure you inhale some of the aromatic steam, too.

YOU WILL NEED

Fresh or dried rosemary
Boiling water
1 teaspoon honey (optional)
Tea strainer

METHOD

Add 2–3 teaspoons of finely chopped rosemary to a tea strainer and pop into a small mug. Pour over boiling water.

Place a saucer over the top of the mug to trap in the aromatics. Leave to infuse for 10–20 minutes, then remove the lid and herbs.

Take a few big deep breaths of the medicinal, rosemary-scented steam and then drink. If you have a sore throat, a spoon of honey can be added to the tea.

TO USE

Drink up to three cups a day.

Rosemary Memory Tincture

If you find it hard to focus your mind, give this brain-boosting herbal tincture a go. Made with brain tonic herbs such as rosemary and stimulating peppermint, it will help blow off the cobwebs. Rosemary is said to promote better blood flow to the brain, which in turn helps to give better mental performance. It also calms the nervous system, making it ideal to take when tackling exams of all types. Avoid if pregnant.

YOU WILL NEED

1 part dried rosemary
1 part dried peppermint
Vodka (at least 40% alcohol)
Clean, dry, wide-mouthed jar with lid
Natural baking parchment
Labels
Muslin (cheesecloth) and fine-mesh strainer
Dropper bottle

METHOD

Finely chop the herbs and half-fill the jar. Use equal parts of each herb. Pour over the vodka, filling the jar.

Place a square of baking parchment over the mouth of the jar, seal and label. Leave to infuse for 4–6 weeks.

Strain into a jug (pitcher) using a strainer lined with a piece of muslin to remove the herbs. Wring out all the liquid.

Funnel this strained liquid into a clean, dry dropper bottle and label. There is no shelf life for an alcohol tincture made with dried herbs, but discard it in the unlikely event that it grows mould or begins to ferment.

TO USE

Take 1–5 ml up to three times a day when required.

Gardener's Ointment for Sore Joints & Muscles

Whether you have an aching back from digging the garden in spring or sore joints in winter, this ointment will help ease any discomfort. Simply massage onto the affected area and place a heat pack on top for additional soothing effects. Comfrey, which we often grow as a green fertiliser/mulch for our garden, is an incredible herb for helping to repair muscles and, interestingly, its folk name is actually 'bone knit'. Combined with warming rosemary, this ointment should be in every gardener's first aid bag.

YOU WILL NEED

For the infused herbal oil:

1 part dried rosemary
2 parts dried comfrey
Your choice of carrier oil, such as olive, rapeseed or sunflower oil

For the ointment:

3 tablespoons rosemary- and comfrey-infused oil
1½ teapoons beeswax pellets
22 drops rosemary essential oil
22 drops ginger essential oil
Double boiler
Small jars or tins with lids
Labels

METHOD

First, make the rosemary- and comfrey-infused herbal oil following the instructions on page 44.

To make the ointment, warm the beeswax over a low heat in a double boiler. Once the wax begins to melt, add 3 tablespoons of the infused oil. Let the wax and oil melt together. Once melted, remove from the heat and stir in the essential oils.

For this recipe, I like to use a 3% dilution of essential oils, which means 22 drops of ginger essential oil and 22 drops of rosemary essential oil, but you should use the correct dilution for your skin (see the Essential Oil Dilution Chart on page 51 for advice on quantities).

Pour the liquid ointment into the jars or tins and seal with a lid. Allow the ointment to cool and harden for 24 hours before labelling and using. The ointment should last approximately 12 months.

TO USE

Simply rub a small amount of the ointment into the area that needs some relief.

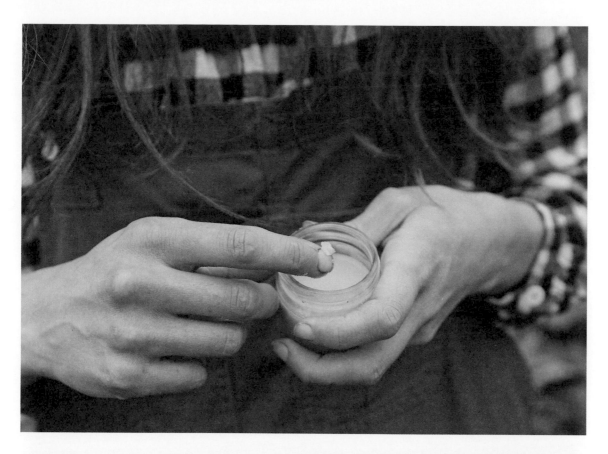

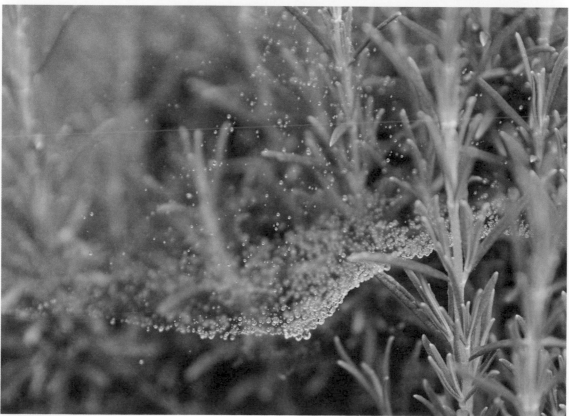

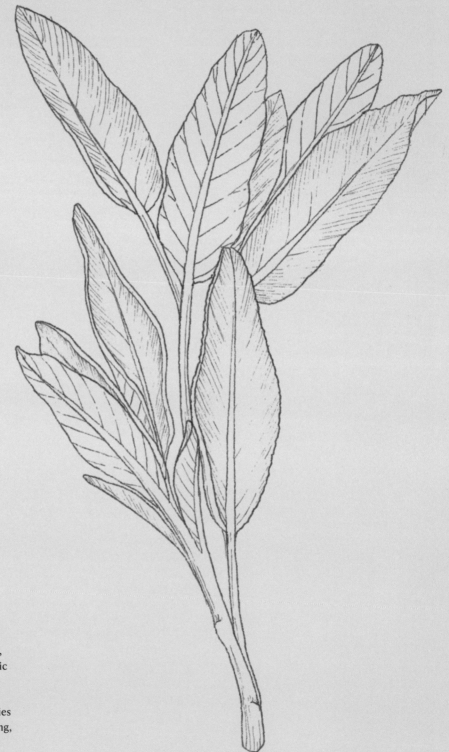

Salvia officinalis

Sage

FAMILY: Lamiaceae

PARTS USED: Leaves

ENERGETICS: Warming and drying

ACTIONS: Antimicrobial, astringent, antispasmodic, diaphoretic, antiseptic and carminative

SAFETY: Do not use in large quantities while pregnant and avoid while nursing, as sage can reduce milk supply.

As a child I was horribly prone to bouts of tonsillitis and so I became very familiar with sage and its abilities to soothe and heal the throat and tonsils. My mum would send me out to harvest a few leaves whenever I felt a sore throat coming on. She'd place the leaves in a cup and pour over boiling water. Once the tea was cool, I'd gargle with the musty-flavoured, aromatic water and feel its benefits soon after.

As I grew out of my childhood illness, I began to discover sage as a delicious culinary herb. I also took it as a tea when I began to wean my children as a way of drying up my milk supply.

Although sage isn't a herb I reach for daily, I feel reassured that I have a pot of this sacred plant steadfastly growing close by.

IDENTIFICATION

Sage is a perennial herb. Its leaves are coated in tiny hairs, giving them a beautiful, velvety texture and slightly grey tinge. The stems are woody and square in shape.

USES

One of the main benefits of sage is its ability to dry and regulate fluids. As I already mentioned, I used sage to help dry up my milk supply when weaning my one year old, but it can also be used to reduce excess sweat (for example, during the menopause) and excessive saliva.

Of course, sage is my choice (alongside thyme) for a sore throat or tonsillitis. Its anti-inflammatory, antimicrobial and antiseptic effects all make it a good option as a strong gargle or throat spray combined with echinacea. It also has decongestant and expectorant qualities that can help ease signs of a cough or bronchitis when taken as a tea or syrup.

Sage is an excellent herb for the mouth. If you suffer with problems such as ulcers, sore gums or general mouth health, you may very well find the astringency of sage alongside its antimicrobial action very soothing and healing. Try using it as a daily gargle in the evenings after brushing your teeth.

Not only is sage delicious as a flavouring for food (I love it on roasted squash), but it also aids the digestion of fats, acts as a digestive system carminative and can ease bloating and gas. Sage is also said to have a protective effect on the liver. Like rosemary, sage can also help boost memory. This is likely due to the anticholinesterase properties of sage, which can in turn support cognitive function, and probably why it is considered a longevity herb. Try sage as part of an uplifting tea blend or use in a tincture for when you need a brain boost.

HARVESTING & PREPARATION

To harvest sage, cut fresh stems and tie them into bunches for drying or, alternatively, dry the leaves in a food dehydrator set at 34°C (93°F) until completely brittle.

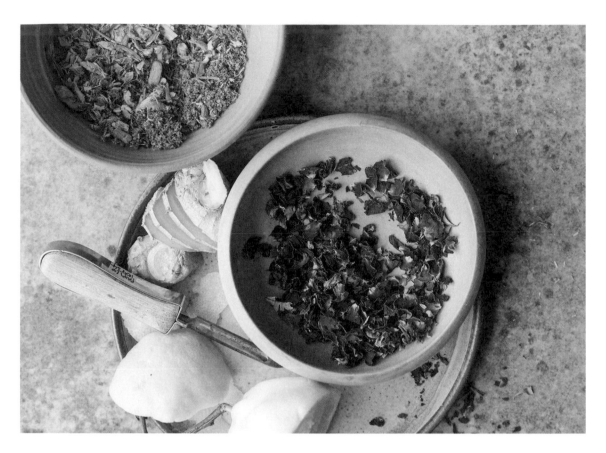

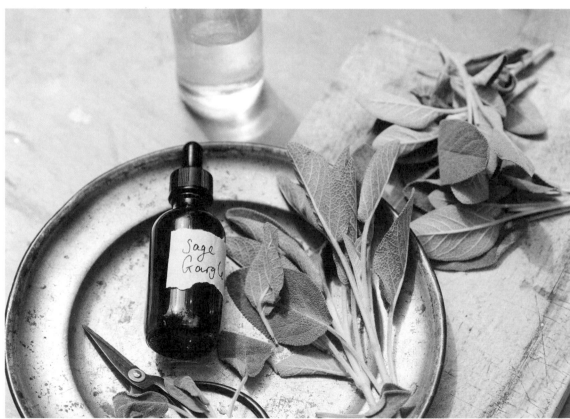

Soothing Throat Tea

As a podcaster I find recording multiple episodes can leave my throat feeling overworked and sounding a bit hoarse. This tea comes to the rescue. I like to brew a large cupful before I settle in front of my microphone and find the soothing effects so welcome. This blend contains marshmallow root which has a high mucilaginous content, giving the tea a slightly gel-like texture that helps to coat and relax the throat.

Ginger and lemon are classic sore throat remedies, while honey, like the marshmallow root, will coat the throat and calm any irritation. The addition of rose gives this tea the perfect floral note, while the astringent qualities can help with swollen tonsils and throat by toning the tissues. You could also use this tea as inspiration for creating a syrup – simply follow the syrup instructions on page 43 and use the ingredients below as a starting point.

YOU WILL NEED

1 teaspoon dried rose petals
1 teaspoon dried marshmallow root
¼ teaspoon dried sage leaves
250 ml (8½ fl oz/1 cup) boiling water
Slice of fresh organic lemon peel
½ teaspoon finely chopped fresh ginger root
1 teaspoon local honey
Teapot

METHOD

Add the herbs, lemon peel and ginger to a teapot and pour over boiling water, making sure all the herbs are fully submerged in the hot water.

Leave the tea to infuse for 10–20 minutes, then remove the herbs. Stir in a teaspoon of honey and drink.

Sage Gargle for Sore Throats

Antiseptic and anti-inflammatory sage makes for the perfect home remedy to help heal scratchy throats. Teamed with some salt, this is my go-to for dealing with the first symptoms.

YOU WILL NEED

Fresh or dried sage, chopped
Strong vodka (at least 40% alcohol)
Clean, dry, wide-mouthed jar with lid
Natural baking parchment
Labels
Muslin (cheesecloth) and fine-mesh strainer
Dropper bottle

METHOD

Make the tincture by filling the jar three-quarters full if using fresh sage and half-full if using dried. Pour over enough vodka to cover the herbs and fill the jar. Stir.

Place a square of baking parchment over the mouth of the jar and seal with the lid.

Label and allow to infuse for 4 weeks.

Strain the finished tincture into a jug (pitcher) using a strainer lined with a piece of muslin to remove the herbs. Funnel into the dropper bottle and label.

Excess tincture can be stored in a labelled bottle.

TO USE

For a quick and powerful throat gargle, add a teaspoon of the tincture and a teaspoon of salt to a small cup of water. Stir well, then gargle and spit out.

Repeat up to three times a day.

Sambucus nigra

Elder

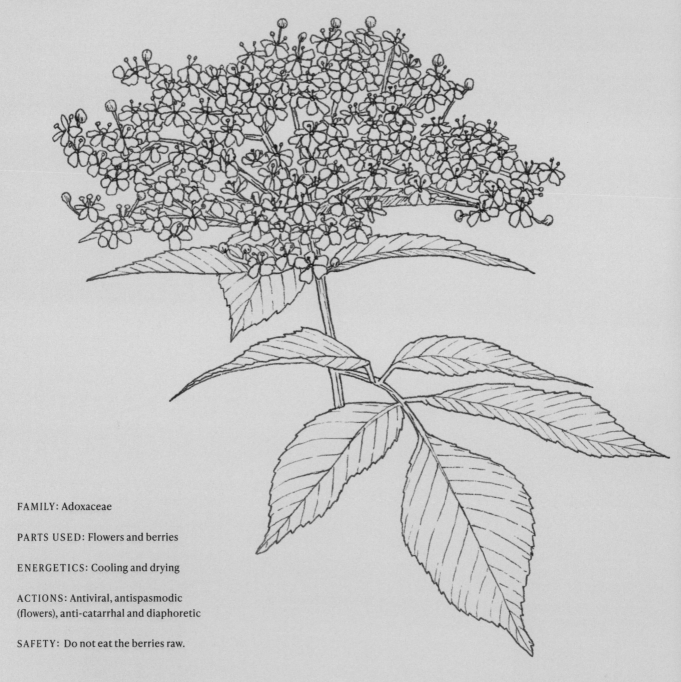

FAMILY: Adoxaceae

PARTS USED: Flowers and berries

ENERGETICS: Cooling and drying

ACTIONS: Antiviral, antispasmodic
(flowers), anti-catarrhal and diaphoretic

SAFETY: Do not eat the berries raw.

Elderflower appears everywhere on the farm in late spring. Along the laneways and in the garden their pretty, umbrella-shaped flower heads herald the arrival of summer and make me dream of sipping elderflower cordial in the garden in the heat of the day.

The unmistakable scent of elders rustles up a half-remembered memory of my annual summer holidays. I can still recall how those little creamy flowers would brush against me on walks along our countryside lanes, leaving powdery pollen on my arms. Later on, in late summer and autumn, the trees would be weighed down with umbrellas of deeply purple, round berries.

Nowadays, I enjoy elderberries cooked into luscious syrups or sauces where they are bursting with health benefits. And, of course, like a lot of people, I consume elderflower profusely in cordials as well as in teas when I'm feeling under the weather.

IDENTIFICATION

Elder is a deciduous shrub with pinnate leaves; there can be 5-7 oval-shaped smaller leaves or leaflets per leaf. These are toothed at the edges.

The flowers are either pale creamy white or pink, depending on the variety, and clustered together in a large, flat umbrella shape. They have a strong and unique scent.

The berries arrive at the end of summer and herald the start of the autumn. They are small, round and dark purple when ripe and hang off the tree in clusters. It is also worth noting that there is a very pretty pink variety of elder called 'Black Lace' which can be used to make a pink-hued cordial.

USES

Although most of us will know and love elderflower cordial, elder actually has many uses beyond being a tasty and traditional summer beverage. The Romans supposedly used elderberries as a hair dye, while their properties have made them a popular herbal remedy for flus and colds. The berries were extensively used in wine making. In fact, there used to be orchards of elder especially for this use.

Elder's berries and flowers have plenty of health benefits due to their vitamin content - mainly A and C - as well as their antiviral, sweat-inducing and anti-allergy effects.

The flowers are often used in a traditional cold and flu tea that is said to have originated from an old gyspy remedy. You can find my version, Gypsy Cold & Flu Syrup, on page 56. Their antiviral properties as well as their ability to regulate a fever make this an important herb. Elderflower is also great for tight, congested sinuses, loosening up mucus and cooling the system. Elderflower combined with nettle leaf is a favourite tea of mine for seasonal allergies and it's also very soothing frozen into an ice pop on hot, pollen-filled days. The flowers of the elder also make a beautiful addition to skincare remedies, due to their ability to encourage healthy blood flow and lower irritation.

There has been some incredible research on elderberries proving that they act as a notable antiviral against the flu virus. The amazing, immune-boosting effects of elderberries make them an essential in my home during cold and flu season. Elderberry can be taken as a honey, tincture or tea, but my favourite way to imbibe them is my Simple Spiced Elderberry Syrup (see page 137).

HARVESTING & PREPARATION

When it comes to picking elderflower, you should pluck the entire umbel of blossoms, not individual flowers, and carefully remove any insects. Pick the flowers on a dry day, preferably at midday, and be careful when handling to ensure as much of the fragrant pollen remains on the flower as possible. Avoid washing the flowers for the same reason and remove any that are brown in colour. Remember to leave some flowers on the tree, so you can pick the berries later on, and also to benefit hungry insects.

Berries are harvested in the same way – by cutting the entire umbrella of berries at the stem – and can be washed. Make sure you toss any green ones away.

Soothing Hay Fever Tea

There's nothing worse than a dose of hay fever with its common symptoms of itchy eyes and runny nose. This tea contains soothing and anti-inflammatory elderflower, plantain and nettle. Ideally, you want to start taking these herbs daily before the onset of the hay fever season as well as during to glean the most benefits. You can also cool the tea, stir in some local honey and freeze in ice pop moulds for a cooling, summer treat.

YOU WILL NEED

Dried nettle leaves
Dried plantain leaves
Dried elderflowers
Boiling water
Local honey (preferably raw)
Airtight jar with lid
Pestle and mortar (optional)
Label
Tea strainer

METHOD

Combine equal parts of nettle leaf, plantain leaf and elderflower in an airtight jar.

Put on the lid and shake to combine. Label the jar.

To make the tea, place 1–3 teaspoons of the herbal tea mix in a tea strainer in your favourite mug. Pour over boiling water.

Let the tea infuse for up to 10–20 minutes. Remove the tea strainer containing the herbs. Stir in a teaspoon of honey and enjoy.

TO USE

Drink up to three cups a day before and throughout the hay fever season.

Botanical Facial Oil

Elderflowers have a long history of being used to perfect the skin and soothing redness and inflammation. In this recipe, I've teamed elderflower with anti-ageing, vitamin C-rich rose hip seed oil to create a beautiful combination that will keep your skin hydrated and nourished. To really boost the power of this recipe, add a few drops of helichrysum essential oil, which has a myriad amazing benefits but is particularly good for aging skin.

YOU WILL NEED

Dried elderflowers (ensure there are no leaves)
Jojoba oil
2 teaspoons rose hip seed oil
6 drops helichrysum essential oil (optional)
Clean, dry, wide-mouthed jar with lid
Fine-mesh strainer
30 ml (1 oz) amber glass dropper bottle
Labels

METHOD

Half-fill the jar with elderflowers. Pour in the jojoba oil until the blooms are completely covered. Give the jar a shake to remove any air pockets, seal tightly with the lid and label. Leave the oil for 4 weeks to infuse, then strain into a jug (pitcher) and discard the elderflowers.

Funnel 20 ml (0.7 oz) of the infused elderflower oil into the dropper bottle alongside the rose hip seed oil. Then add the helichrysum essential oil.

Seal the bottle with the lid, shake gently to combine and then label. The oil will last about 12 months.

TO USE

Place a few drops of oil on your palms, apply over cleansed skin and finish with your favourite face cream. The oil can be used morning and night.

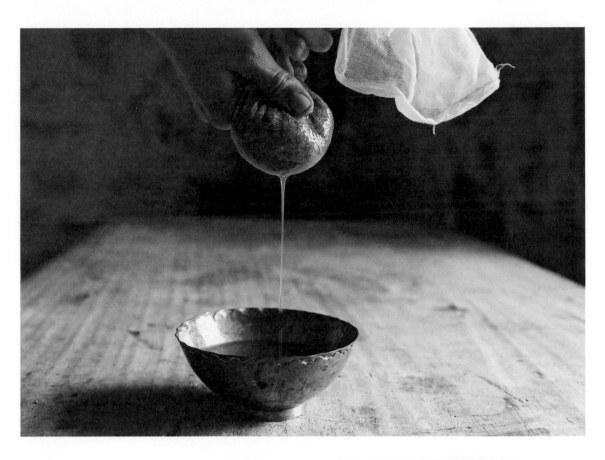

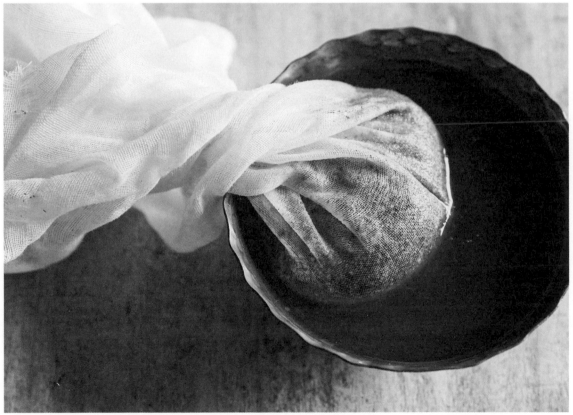

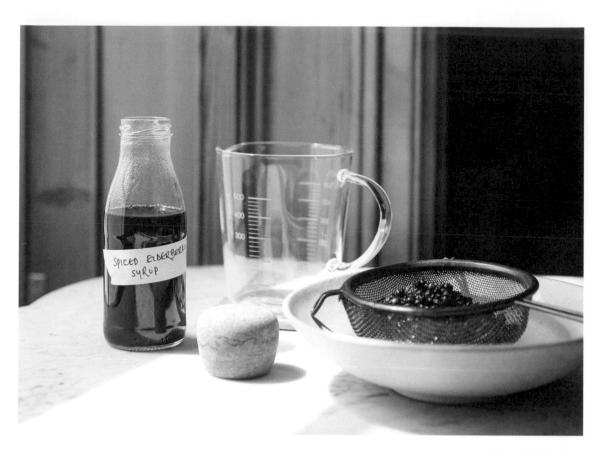

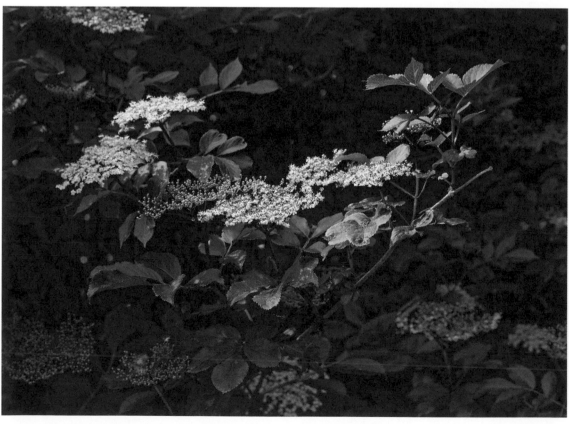

Simple Spiced Elderberry Syrup

Elderberry syrup is a classic recipe for the home apothecary. It is perfect for boosting the immune system and helping to ward off unwanted colds and flu. I love the addition of some warming and antimicrobial spices such as ginger, clove and cinnamon to add more flavour and health benefits.

YOU WILL NEED

125 g (4 oz) fresh or dried elderberries
500 ml (16 fl oz/2 cups) water
62–125 g (2–4 oz/½–1 cup) plain or elderberry-infused honey (see page 41 for how to make a herbal honey)
1 cinnamon stick
6 whole cloves
2½ cm (1 in) piece of fresh ginger root, thinly sliced
1 tablespoon elderberry tincture (optional) (see page 47 for how to make a tincture)
Muslin (cheesecloth) and fine-mesh strainer
Storage bottle with lid
Label

METHOD

Begin by washing the fresh berries and removing and discarding the stems and leaves. If you are using dried berries, then skip this step.

Place the berries, cinnamon stick, cloves and ginger in a saucepan and add the water. Bring to the boil and then simmer until the berries are completely soft and the water has reduced by about half. Allow to cool slightly, then strain into a jug (pitcher).

You should have about 250 ml (8½ fl oz/1 cup) of liquid left at this point. If you have too much, you can return the liquid to the heat to reduce further. If too much water has evaporated, add a little more to make it up to one cup.

Add the honey, stir well to combine and then funnel into a bottle and label. If necessary, you can warm the herbal liquid and honey together in the saucepan to combine them.

Keep refrigerated and use within 4 weeks.

Variation

You can add a tablespoon of elderberry tincture or brandy to improve the shelf life of the syrup. Add this right at the end before bottling and stir in well. Using the elderberry tincture has the advantage of adding even more elderberry power!

TO USE

Take 1 tablespoon once a day during the autumn and winter months. Children over the age of one can have 1 teaspoon a day during the cold and flu season. I also love a spoon of this syrup mixed into warm water as a comforting drink when I have the sniffles.

Stellaria media

Chickweed

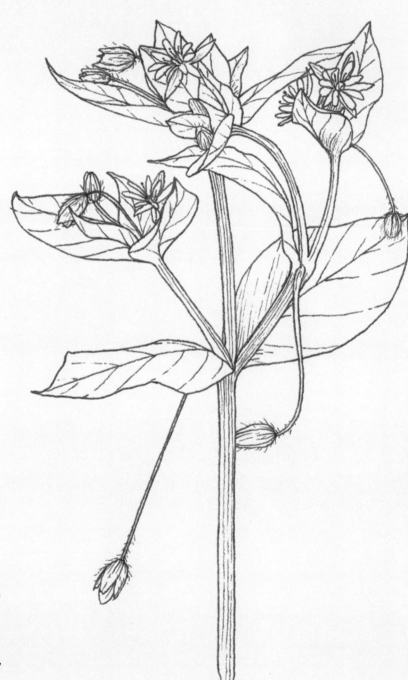

FAMILY: Caryophyllaceae

PARTS USED: Aerial parts

ENERGETICS: Cooling and moistening

ACTIONS: Anti-inflammatory, alterative,
antirheumatic, demulcent, diuretic,
emollient, vulnerary and nutritive

Chickweed grows almost uncontrollably here at the farm. It envelopes our vegetable patch in summer and carpets the garden beds if given half a chance. Even in winter it keeps growing in our polytunnels!

My discovery of chickweed's herbal uses coincided with my eldest son getting a bad bout of infant eczema. I had tried absolutely everything to little effect and was desperate to find a way to soothe his skin and heal the sore cracked patches. It was then that I came across chickweed quite by chance (as is often the way with herbs, they appear just when you need them!). Learning about the calming properties of chickweed, I decided to try making my own gentle chickweed balm. It worked and from that I have gone on to use chickweed in many ways.

So, instead of popping chickweed onto the compost heap, put it in your garden trug and take it back to your kitchen and try some of the following recipes.

IDENTIFICATION

Chickweed's most identifiable feature is the single line of hairs that run along each stem. This makes for a quick and easy way of making sure you have the right plant! Other important things to note are its pretty, white, star-like flowers (hence the Latin name *stellaria*). There is a visually similar plant to chickweed called scarlet pimpernel (*Anagallis arvensis*), which has red flowers and is toxic, so should be avoided.

USES

Chickweed is a very nutritious weed and considered a good addition to the diet of anyone in need of a nutritional boost. Chickweed is nutrient-rich, containing plenty of beneficial minerals and vitamins A and C. It was revered in the past as a green for strengthening those that were run down or convalescing. Chickweed's cooling and anti-inflammatory qualities are also helpful for a range of digestive issues.

While it can be sautéed in a pan like spinach, I prefer it made into a pesto. I often grab a handful when I'm out in the garden and blitz it up with some Parmesan, garlic and oil for a tasty accompaniment at lunchtime. If you love a daily green juice, you could try chickweed in it, too. Chickweed is at its best when its growth is still young and when the shoots are still tender, so avoid harvesting from older plants that are going to seed.

Chickweed is a wonderful herb for sore, itchy, eczema-prone skin. Its anti-inflammatory, cooling and moistening effects help to calm the skin and aid healing. Try a chickweed balm or, alternatively, make a strong chickweed tea and add this to your bath water to soothe the skin. For minor cuts, grazes, rashes and so on a poultice made with chickweed and chamomile can give instant relief and help promote healing. This combination of herbs can also be used as a compress for irritated eyes (see my Chickweed & Chamomile Compress on page 143).

Chickweed has also been known to help shift benign cysts and lipomas successfully. This is likely due to the high saponin content of the herb. Saponins help the body to break down fatty deposits and encourage healthy mucus membranes. A fresh chickweed tincture applied externally or taken internally is a possible remedy to explore, although it is important to go to a doctor to rule out any more serious issues first. Overall, chickweed is a herb to reach for to nourish and to help cool and lubricate the system and bring balance to the water levels in the body.

HARVESTING & PREPARATION

If you are weeding chickweed, pull it up by the roots and carefully snip these off, trying to stop any soil getting into the shoots and leaves. Otherwise, just harvest like a cut-and-come-again salad leaf and snip off the fresh shoots close to the ground, leaving the roots in the soil. Look for lush young plants that have juicy stems.

Chickweed can be dried laid out on a basket or in a food dehydrator set at about 37°C (99°F).

Gentle Chickweed & Borage Balm

This balm is one of the recipes in the book that I use the most. It's so effective at soothing and calming sore and sensitive skin and has helped calm down my eldest son's eczema. If you don't have time to make the infused chickweed oil in the first part of the recipe, you can purchase this to speed up the process (see Resources on page 174 for a recommended supplier). Borage seed oil helps to reduce inflammation and is said to have a regenerative effect on the skin.

YOU WILL NEED

For the chickweed-infused oil:

Dried chickweed
Sunflower or olive oil
Clean, dry, wide-mouthed jar with lid
Labels
Muslin (cheesecloth) and fine-mesh strainer
Storage bottle with lid

For the balm:

1 tablespoon beeswax pellets
2 tablespoons infused chickweed oil
1 tablespoon borage seed oil
85g (3 oz) shea butter, roughly chopped
5 drops German chamomile (*Matricaria recutita*) essential oil
Double boiler
Small jar or tin with lid
Label

METHOD

Fill a jar half-full with dried chickweed.

Pour over sunflower or olive oil until the chickweed is completely covered. Seal the jar with the lid, then label. Allow to infuse for 4 weeks, then strain the liquid into a jug (pitcher) using a strainer lined with a piece of muslin to remove the plant material. Funnel into a bottle and you now have a chickweed-infused oil.

The oil can now be used as a calming chickweed body oil, but I like to turn it into a balm for easier use.

To make the balm, melt the beeswax pellets over a low heat in a double boiler. Once the beeswax has started to melt, add the infused chickweed oil, the borage seed oil and shea butter, and stir until all the wax has melted and you have a liquid.

Remove from the heat and stir in the German chamomile essential oil. (This will turn the balm a pale shade of blue due to the high chamazulene content in the essential oil.) Pour the balm into a small jar or tin and seal with the lid. Allow to cool and harden for 24 hours before labelling and using.

The balm should last for 12 months. If you are using a fresh chickweed infusion, you may find the balm has a shorter shelf life.

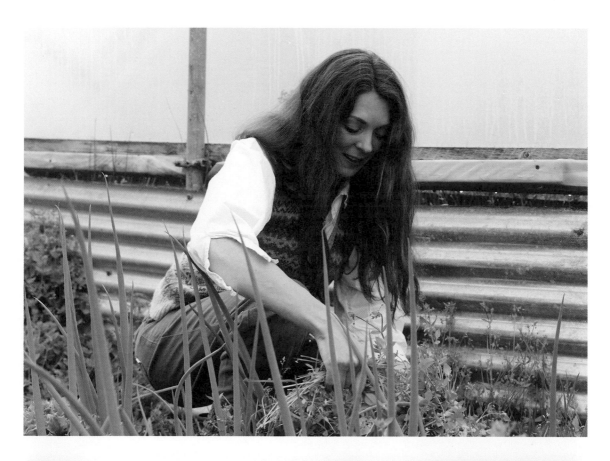

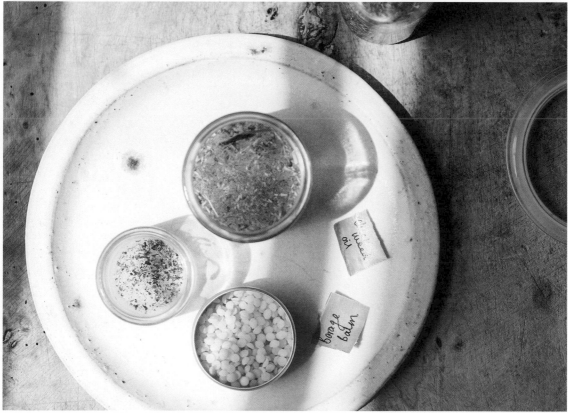

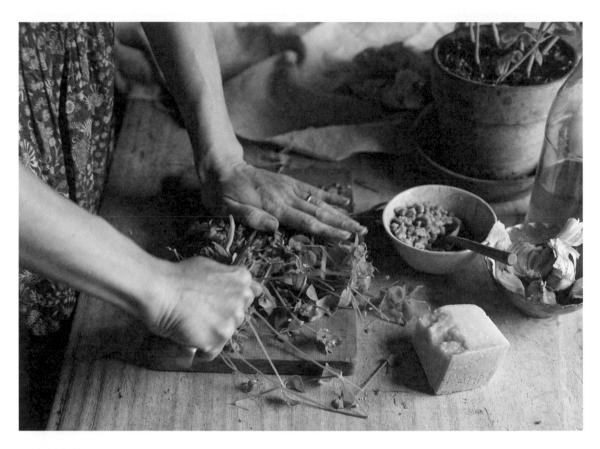

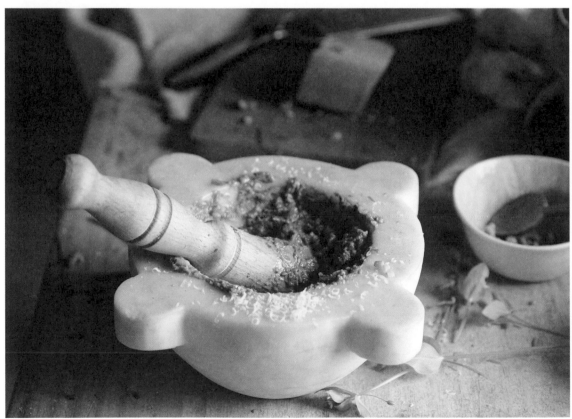

Chickweed Pesto

This is one of my favourite recipes to rustle up throughout the year. It makes the most out of the abundant chickweed that thrives in our polytunnels and garden beds and gives the body a boost, thanks to the nutrient- and mineral-rich chickweed. The key to making this pesto super delicious is to use a basil-infused extra-virgin olive oil. This is easy to make at home. Just fill a bottle one-third full with some dried basil and top with olive oil. Strain after four weeks and you have the perfect oil for making any pesto!

YOU WILL NEED

100 g (3½ oz) wild edible greens (in this case, chickweed)
50 g (2 oz) good-quality walnuts
200 ml (7 fl oz/scant 1 cup) basil-infused extra-virgin olive oil
   (see page 44 for how to make an infused oil)
40 g (1½ oz) finely grated Parmesan cheese
1–2 garlic cloves
Salt and freshly ground black pepper

METHOD

Add the edible greens (here, I've used chickweed) to a food processor with the walnuts, olive oil, Parmesan cheese and garlic. Blend until almost smooth and season to taste.

Use in sandwiches, stirred through pasta and even as the base of a salad dressing. Delicious!

Chickweed & Chamomile Compress

This compress can provide wonderful relief, whether your tired or irritated eyes are thanks to seasonal allergies, wearing contact lenses or too much screen time. Chamomile is antimicrobial, anti-inflammatory and soothing, while chickweed is cooling, moistening and also has anti-inflammatory properties.

YOU WILL NEED

1 tablespoon chopped fresh chickweed
1 tablespoon fresh or dried chamomile flowers
200 ml (7 fl oz/1 cup) boiling water
¼ teaspoon salt
Muslin (cheesecloth) and fine-mesh strainer
Clean cloth or cotton-wool pad

METHOD

Add the chickweed and chamomile to a bowl. Pour over the boiling water, sprinkle in the salt and leave to infuse for 20 minutes.

Strain the liquid into a clean, dry bowl using a strainer lined with a piece of muslin to remove the herbs.

TO USE

Once the herbal liquid is cool enough, soak a clean cloth or cotton-wool pad in it. Wring it out and place over your closed eye(s). Leave on the eyes for around 5 minutes. Repeat as needed, using a fresh cloth each time. Extra liquid can be kept in the fridge for 24 hours.

Taraxacum officinale

Dandelion

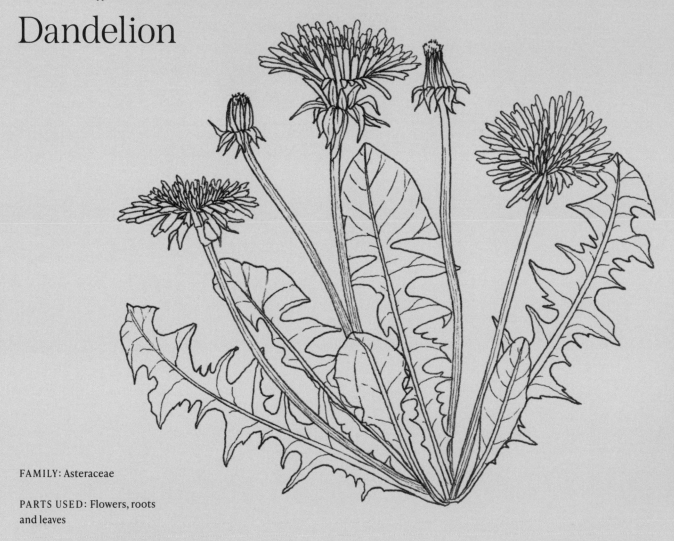

FAMILY: Asteraceae

PARTS USED: Flowers, roots
and leaves

ENERGETICS: Cooling and drying

ACTIONS: Hepatic, nutritive,
bitter, diuretic, cholagogue (root)
and laxative

SAFETY: Avoid if allergic to the
Asteraceae family and consult a
GP if you have any gallbladder, liver
or kidney concerns before using.

To me, dandelions are synonymous with childhood. Who hasn't played clocks with the fluffy ripe seed heads? Or marvelled at their bright yellow flowers? Like many of my favourite childhood plants, dandelion came into my kitchen much later on when I became interested in herbalism. I was surprised to learn that dandelion wasn't just a tenacious and tough weed, and it soon became a regular spring green in my cooking. The taste of dandelion's bitter leaves, the honeyed blossoms and strong root are all flavours I enjoy immensely, and their bright, cheery, yellow flowers dotted about on my lawn are very welcome. Dandelions are also an important food source for pollinators such as bees, being one of the earliest spring flowers.

IDENTIFICATION

Dandelions are a hugely abundant perennial herb, although some would call them a weed. When it comes to identifying dandelions, their leaves are long, hairless and irregularly lobed. It is thought that these toothed leaves are the reason for the French name *dent-de-lion*, meaning 'teeth of the lion'. The leaves of dandelions come directly from the basal rosette (that is, right at the base of the plant near the ground). The stems are quite thick and hollow, producing a white sap when broken. Each stem has one bright yellow flower on top, which is large in size with multiple thin petals. These flowers open and close with the sun and will go to seed after about four days from first flowering.

USES

Dandelions are a respected salad leaf in many countries, used in pasties and salads and even grown in complete darkness to create a pale and milder tasting leaf. They are a brilliant medicinal herb for the liver and can be used as a digestive tonic as well. Dandelions are rich in iron, full of potassium, and vitamins A and C and are a great addition to our diets, especially after a long winter when we are in need of a digestive boost. My favourite way of consuming the young spring leaves is by sautéeing them in ghee. This tempers out the bitter flavour and tastes incredible!

Dandelion leaves are highly beneficial as a safe and very effective diuretic which can be used to combat water retention. They help to increase urination but do so in a gentle way that also provides essential potassium. Dandelion leaves can be eaten fresh, infused in vinegar (see my recipe for Spring Greens Vinegar on page 165), as a tea or tinctured.

Dandelion root has cleansing and detoxifying properties as a hepatic (otherwise known as a liver-protecting herb). It is said that dandelion root can stimulate the liver and bile production, which in turn can be good for certain joint and skin issues. My favourite way of consuming dandelion root is in a roasted coffee alternative (see Dandelion Roasted Coffee, page 148). It gives me great pleasure to sit in my garden and raise a cup of hot dandelion coffee to my freshly weeded garden.

The dandelion root is also a source of iron and is often used by herbalists in conjunction with yellow dock (*Rumex crispus*) for treating anaemia. Young spring roots can be used to flavour salads and are good sliced very finely.

As for the sunshine yellow dandelion flowers, they can be battered and eaten as fritters, infused into syrups, used as decoration for salads and cakes, and the buds can be pickled. They can also be fermented to create wine.

HARVESTING & PREPARATION

The roots are best harvested in autumn. Dig around the root carefully to stop breakage and wash thoroughly. Once sliced thinly, it can be dried on trays in a warm, dry place or in a food dehydrator set at 40°C (104°F). The leaves are best harvested in spring when they are still young and not too bitter. Older leaves are better left to tinctures. The flowers can be harvested throughout spring and summer.

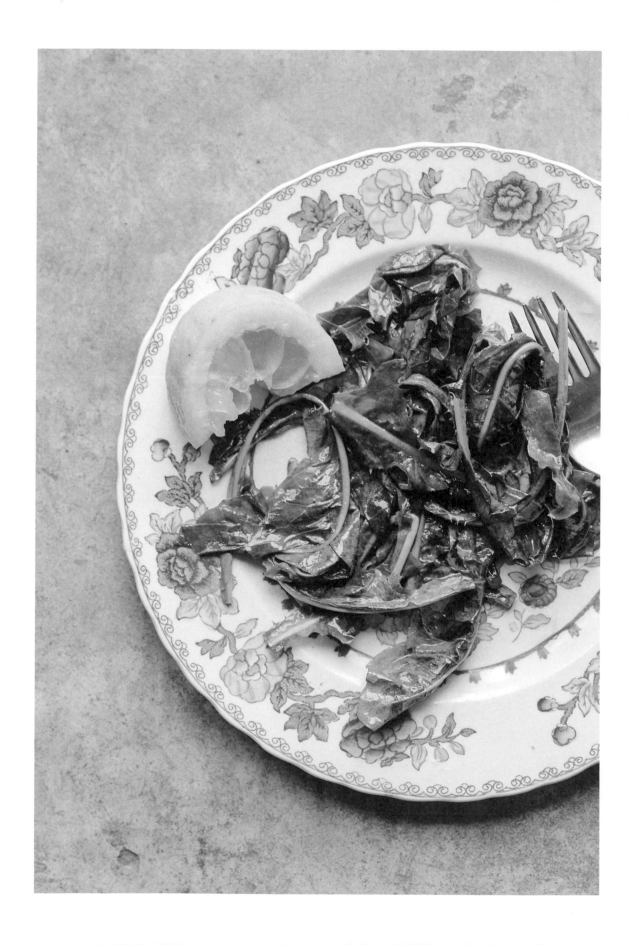

Sautéed Dandelion Greens

While dandelion greens are bitter, they also taste delicious when sautéed with plenty of butter or olive oil. Young dandelion greens are a great source of valuable nutrients, have cleansing properties, and are one of my favourite spring greens to eat!

YOU WILL NEED

Handful of freshly picked young dandelion leaves, washed, dried and chopped into thirds
1 garlic clove, crushed
Butter or organic olive oil
Salt and freshly ground black pepper

METHOD

Heat some butter or olive oil in a frying pan (skillet) over a medium heat. Add the garlic and sauté lightly until soft.

Add the dandelion greens to the pan and sauté until cooked through. This will take about 2-3 minutes.

Season to taste with salt and black pepper and add a knob of extra butter or a drizzle of olive oil. Add a squeeze of lemon juice if desired.

Spring Tonic Tea

This grounding, green-hued tea will certainly wake you up after a long winter. The nettle provides nutrients and prepares the body for the allergy season, while cleavers support the lymphatic system and dandelion root helps the liver. The flavour is mild and earthy with an invigorating mint note, making it a wonderful daytime drink. You can add a spoon of local raw honey, too, if you like a touch of sweetness.

YOU WILL NEED

1 teaspoon dried nettle leaves
½ teaspoon dried cleavers (aerial parts)
¼ teaspoon dried dandelion root
½ teaspoon dried peppermint leaves
Boiling water
Tea strainer

METHOD

Place the nettle leaves, cleavers, dandelion root and peppermint leaves in a tea strainer.

Put the strainer inside a mug and pour over boiling water, ensuring all the herbs are submerged completely.

Allow to infuse for 10 minutes, then remove the herbs in the strainer and enjoy.

Dandelion Roasted Coffee

This tasty coffee alternative came about when I needed a caffeine-free option during pregnancy. It soon became a firm favourite and now we serve it up in our farm café, too! The dandelion and chicory in this recipe are wonderful for supporting the liver, perfect for a healthier morning brew.

YOU WILL NEED

1 part fresh or dried dandelion roots
1 part fresh or dried chicory roots
½ part cocoa nibs
Food dehydrator (optional)
Airtight jars with lids
Coffee grinder or food processor
Label

METHOD

If you are using dandelion and chicory roots that are already dried, you can skip the first few stages. If you are using fresh roots, then wash them thoroughly, pat dry with some paper towel and chop into matchsticks.

Allow the roots to dry for 24 hours on trays in a warm, dry room, keeping the dandelion and chicory separate.

At this point you can either pop the roots in a food dehydrator set at about 42°C (108°F) or leave them to continue drying on their trays.

Preheat the oven to 180°C/350°F/gas 4 (reducing the temperature to 160°C/320°F/gas 4 for a fan oven). Spread the dried dandelion roots out on a flat baking sheet. Put the dried chicory roots in a dry, airtight jar.

Roast the dried dandelion roots in the oven for about 20 minutes or until they turn a roasted brown colour. Remove from the oven and allow to cool.

In a coffee grinder or food processor, pulse the dried roots (keeping the chicory and dandelion separate) until roughly chopped. Repeat with the cocoa nibs.

Now it's time to blend the coffee. Add 1 part of roasted dandelion root and 1 part of dried chicory root to a jar. Sprinkle in the ground cocoa nibs. Stir and label the jar with the contents and date.

TO USE

Add 1 teaspoon of the mixture to a tea infuser or strainer and pour over boiling water in a mug. Infuse for a couple of minutes. Remove the infuser or strainer. Enjoy!

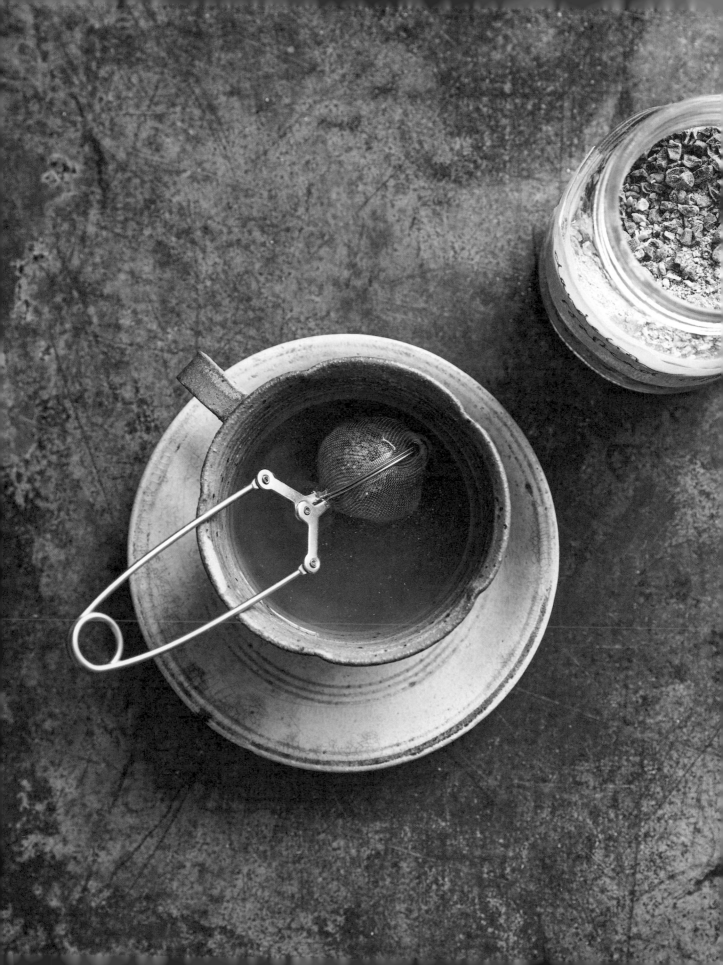

Thymus vulgaris

Thyme

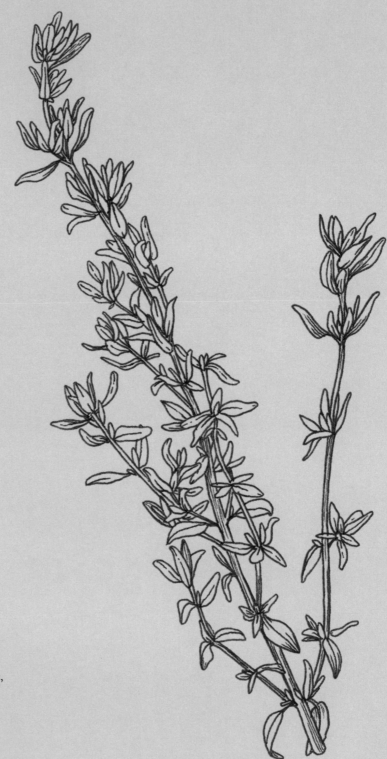

FAMILY: Lamiaceae

PARTS USED: Leaves

ENERGETICS: Warming and drying

ACTIONS: Antimicrobial, antispasmodic, astringent, carminative, digestive and expectorant

SAFETY: Do not use thyme in large quantities while pregnant.

It probably says a lot that the first container you come across when you open my cottage door is one that's full of thyme. Thyme is such a dependable and classic herb. It goes into my stock pot weekly, is sprinkled liberally over all my roasts and is infused into teas when I feel chesty or have a sore throat coming on. I even use the essential oil (thymus linalool) diluted in some sunflower oil for an immune boost when I feel a cold stirring.

Even better, thyme hangs on in there, even through the nastiest of frosts, and doesn't panic if I forget to water it (which I admit does happen quite often!). So, it keeps my kitchen stocked with a fresh fragrant herb throughout the year and happens to be the perfect remedy for the whole family, too.

IDENTIFICATION

Thyme is a low-growing perennial that thrives in full sun and dry conditions. It has tiny leaves arranged opposite each other on the stem. Older stems have a woody appearance.

USES

If you find yourself getting upper respiratory issues such as a cold, chesty cough, infections or sore throat, thyme could be the herb for you. It has antimicrobial, expectorant and warming effects that help to loosen stuck mucus and could help fight off stubborn infections. This is likely due to its strengthening effect on the thymus gland, which in turn boosts immunity and helps fight infection. A cup of honey-sweetened thyme tea is an easy and effective way of benefitting from this herb.

A thyme herbal steam is also an effective home remedy for bronchitis. It will also open tight sinuses, help aid healing and provide relief from heavy head colds and sinus issues. Try the Opening Herbal Steam recipe on page 154 next time you feel congested and in need of relief.

Thyme is one of the best herbs for sore throats, mouths and gums. A strong thyme infusion, allowed to cool and used as a gargle, can help with general mouth health and keep tonsils clean and healthy, too, thanks to the antimicrobial qualities of the herb. For a sore throat, try taking an oxymel, infused honey or thyme syrup. This will coat the throat and also deliver some of the amazing health benefits of thyme.

Other important uses of thyme are as a helpful digestive herb, thanks to its high volatile oil content. Thyme can help ease uncomfortable bloating, a sore stomach or aid healing from a tummy bug. It can also effectively disinfect and clean minor wounds when used as a wash.

HARVESTING & PREPARATION

Cut lengths of the leafy stems (flowers are okay!) and tie into bunches for drying or, alternatively, dry the leaves in a food dehydrator set at 34°C (93°F) until completely brittle and dry.

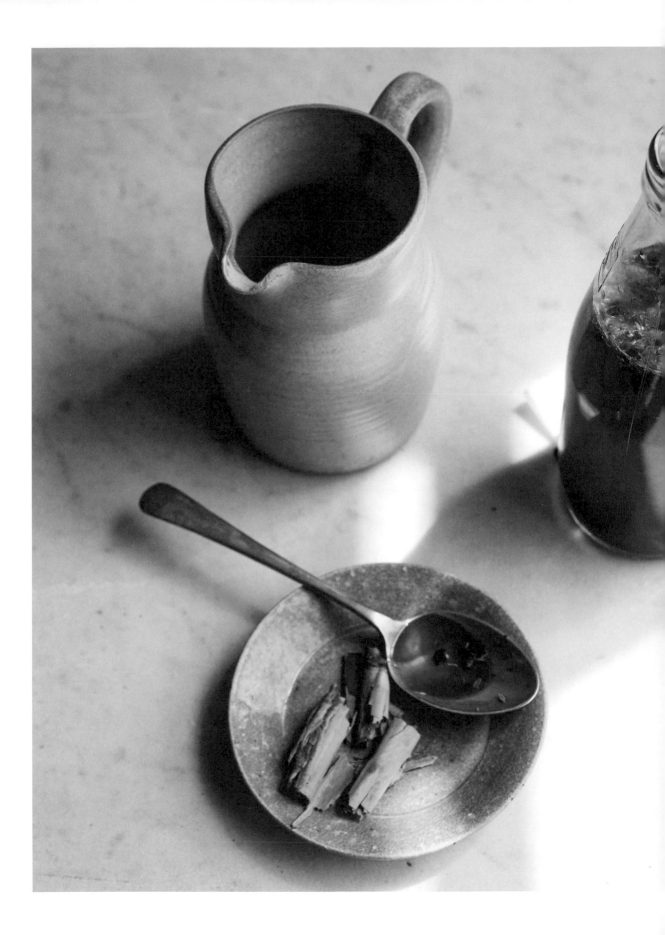

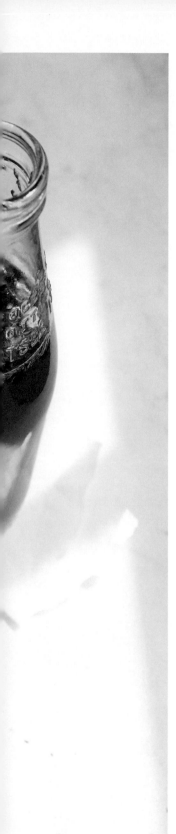

Thyme & Elderberry Oxymel

Oxymels are a delicious way of enjoying plant medicine. Vinegar extracts the medicinal properties and honey provides a delicious sweetness and coats the throat. Take a teaspoon daily or up to 3 teaspoons when you're feeling under the weather. This recipe is also tasty when a spoonful is added to warm water, which in turn keeps the system hydrated. This oxymel is safe for children but avoid giving to babies under the age of one.

YOU WILL NEED

1 part dried thyme (aerial parts)
1 part dried elderberries
1 cinnamon stick, crushed
2.5 cm (1 in) piece of fresh ginger root, finely diced
Raw apple cider vinegar
Raw honey
Clean, dry, wide-mouthed jar with lid
Natural baking parchment
Labels
Muslin (cheesecloth) and fine-mesh strainer
Storage bottle with lid

METHOD

Half-fill the jar with the thyme, elderberries and spices. Fill the jar half-full with apple cider vinegar. Top up the jar to the shoulder point with honey and stir well.

Place a square of baking parchment over the mouth of the jar, seal with the lid and label. Allow the herbs to infuse into the vinegar and honey liquid for around 4 weeks. I like to give the jar a shake occasionally in order to keep the infusion awake and active.

When the oxymel is ready, strain into a jug (pitcher) using a strainer lined with a piece of muslin to remove the herbs. Funnel into the bottle and label.

TO USE

Take 1–3 teaspoons a day or dilute in warm water for a hot drink.

Thyme, Elecampane & Ginger Cough Syrup

This effective cough syrup will help support the respiratory system and ease the symptoms of coughs and colds. Thyme is particularly suited to damp, wet coughs with plenty of mucus. This syrup has warming and expectorant qualities that should give relief from a persistent cough. Elecampane is an excellent herb for the lungs and will help shift any stuck mucus (it can be bought online).

YOU WILL NEED

95 g (3½ oz/¾ cup) dried thyme (aerial parts)
32 g (1½ oz/¼ cup) dried elecampane root
2½ cm (1 in) piece of fresh ginger root, finely chopped
500 ml (16 fl oz/2 cups) water
62–125 g (2–4 oz/½–1 cup) honey or sugar
2 tablespoons brandy
Muslin (cheesecloth) and fine-mesh strainer
Storage bottle with lid
Label

METHOD

Add the herbs, ginger and water to a saucepan. Bring to the boil and simmer very gently for 20 minutes, until half the water has evaporated. Cool and strain.

Return the liquid to the pan. If too much water has evaporated, add more to make the quantity up to 250 ml (8½ fl oz/1 cup). Add the honey or sugar. Stir well to combine. If using sugar, simmer until dissolved completely.

Cool slightly and add the brandy. Stir well and then funnel the syrup into the bottle. Label and refrigerate. Use within 4 weeks.

TO USE

Take 1–3 teaspoons when needed.

Opening Herbal Steam

Next time you're feeling sniffly and congested, give this plant-packed steam a go. It contains herbs that clear and help decongest the sinuses as well as delivering antibacterial properties.

YOU WILL NEED

1 tablespoon chopped fresh or dried thyme (aerial parts)
1 tablespoon chopped fresh or dried rosemary (aerial parts)
1 tablespoon chopped fresh or dried sage (aerial parts)
1 tablespoon chopped fresh or dried peppermint (aerial parts)
Couple of drops peppermint or eucalyptus essential oil
    (optional, as these are not suitable for children)
Boiling water

METHOD

Mix all the herbs together in a large bowl and pour over just-boiled water. Add the peppermint essential oil, if using.

Carefully lower your head toward the bowl, being careful not to get too close – you want to be near enough to be able to inhale the aromatic healing steam but not close enough to get overheated.

Put a large towel over your head, enveloping yourself in a DIY steam room. Allow yourself around 5–7 minutes to inhale the aromatics deeply.

When you have finished, pour the now-cooled water over any plants (they love that herbal water, too!). Discard the herbs in the compost bin.

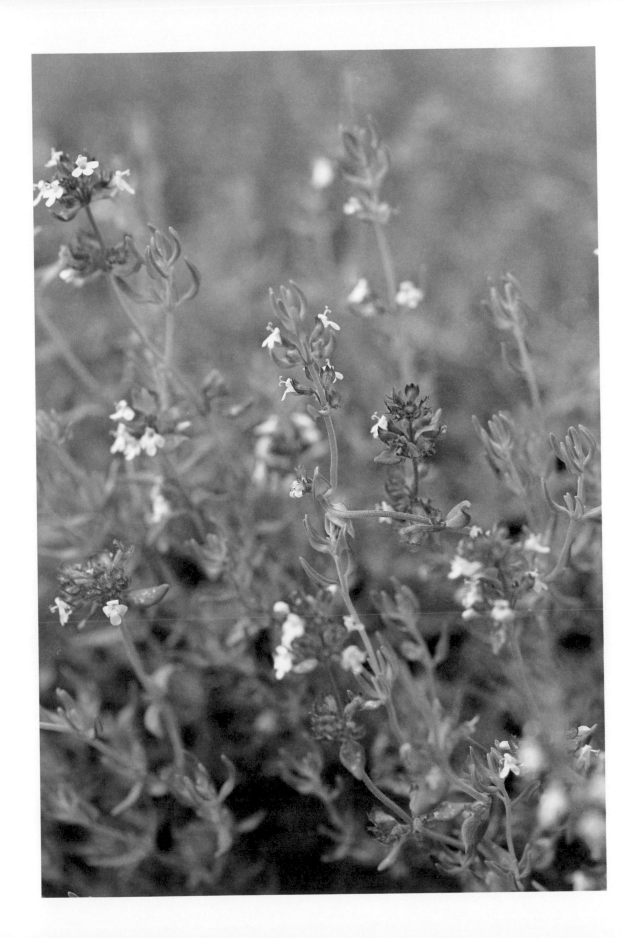

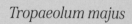
Tropaeolum majus

Nasturtium

FAMILY: Tropaeolaceae

PARTS USED: Leaves, flowers and seeds

ENERGETICS: Warming

ACTIONS: Antibacterial, antibiotic, antifungal, antitussive, cholagogue, disinfectant, diuretic and expectorant

SAFETY: In general, nasturtium is safe, but caution is required if pregnant or nursing.

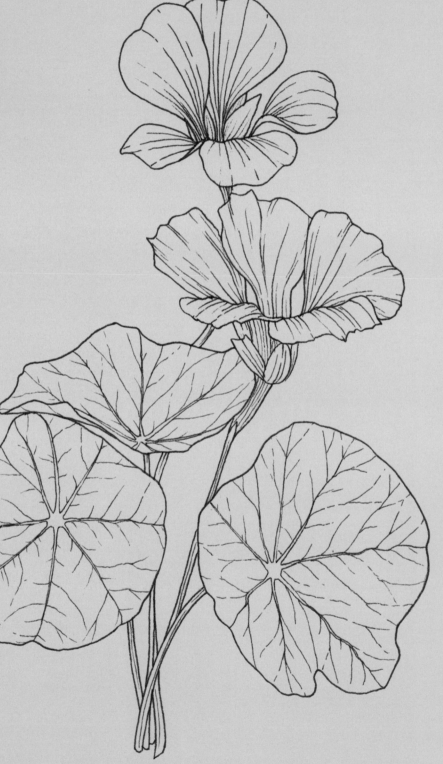

I'm a huge advocate of growing edible flowers and using them prolifically during the summer on cakes for our farm shop or in salads and infusions. Of the many I grow here I always get excited when I see the return of the vivid nasturtium. Their beautiful and intricate flowers have long held a fascination for me. As a child I loved to find the sweet nectar hidden in the spur of the flower, a stolen treat before supper. And I still enjoy snacking on their blossoms during summer when I'm working in the garden.

Nasturtiums are often used as a decorative addition to flower beds or in containers, which is how I like to grow mine. I even put them in my window boxes. Apart from bringing a great splash of colour and being a useful aphid trap (aphids flock to nasturtiums, often sparing other plants), nasturtiums are really quite delicious and, of course, medicinal!

IDENTIFICATION

Nasturtiums have almost round leaves with prominent pale veins and are attached in the middle of the leaf to long, juicy stems. The trumpet-like flowers come in shades of red and yellow but more unusual varieties are now also available.

USES

Apart from their delicious peppery flavour, nasturtiums are also a great support for the respiratory system. Their expectorant, antibiotic and antibacterial qualities and vitamin C content make them a useful plant for relieving colds and upper respiratory infections. Try diluting a nasturtium flower vinegar with some honey and warm water as a soothing remedy for a bothersome cold or cough or try the Nasturtium & Orange Oxymel (see page 160).

Nasturtium leaves and flowers can be applied topically to help heal and disinfect minor cuts or mild fungal infections. The best way of doing this is to create a poultice by mashing up some leaves and flowers and applying this over the area, using a thin bandage between the skin and herb if necessary.

The flowers, leaves and seeds are all wonderful used in the kitchen. Peppery, spicy and even a little sweet thanks to the nectar, the flowers are a very welcome addition when used fresh in any salad or chopped and folded into butter. The leaves can be shredded and used as a salad leaf, in savoury tarts and in omelettes. The seeds are wonderful pickled and eaten the same way as capers. The stimulating effects of nasturtium help to promote good digestion while the bitter quality helps liver function and increases elimination, making it a wonderful kitchen herb for summer.

HARVESTING & PREPARATION

Harvest the flowers throughout summer and use them fresh or preserve them in vinegar. The leaves can be used fresh but can be dried, too, either on a tray in a warm, dry room or in a food dehydrator set at about 37°C (99°F). Keep drying the leaves until they are completely crisp and dry, then store in a dry, airtight jar. Seeds are best pickled. Otherwise, they can be dried and used for sowing the following year.

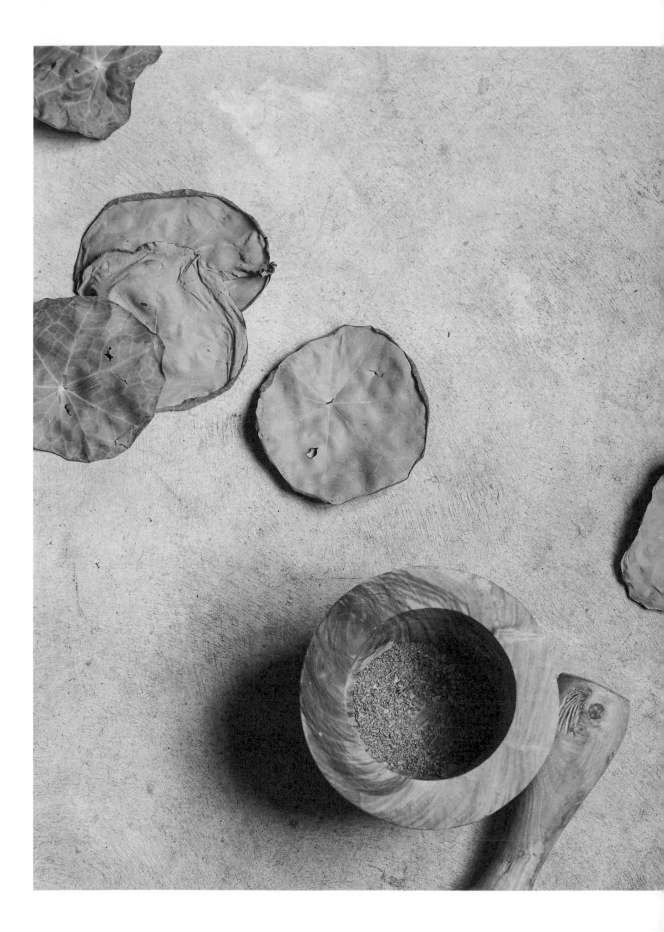

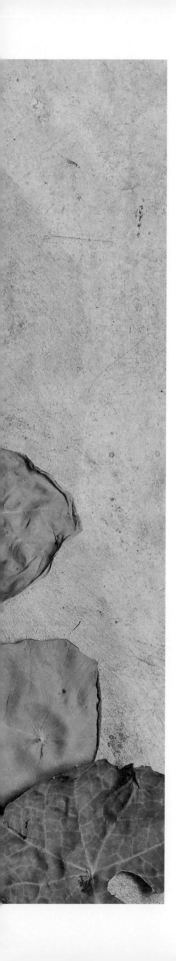

Nasturtium Leaf Sprinkle

Harness some of the amazing properties of nasturtiums in this tasty seasoning. Sprinkle over any dish that needs a spicy kick.

YOU WILL NEED

Dried nasturtium leaves
Salt
Pepper
Drying rack or food dehydrator
Pestle and mortar or food processor
Spice container
Label

METHOD

Harvest a handful of nasturtium leaves. Dry the leaves on a drying rack or in a food dehydrator until completely dry.

Blitz up the leaves, either using a pestle and mortar or in a food processor. Then, for every tablespoon of ground nasturtium, add ¼ teaspoon of salt and ¼ teaspoon of pepper.

Mix well, pour into a clean, dry spice container and label. Sprinkle over food as a seasoning.

Nasturtium Seed Capers

Sometimes known as poor man's capers, these are a great way of using up excess seeds from summer's nasturtiums. The spicy flavour will be sure to open up the airways.

YOU WILL NEED

Freshly picked nasturtium seeds
500 ml (16 fl oz/2 cups) water
30 g (1 oz) salt
Clean, dry, wide-mouthed jar with lid
Fine-mesh strainer

For the pickling liquid:

150 g (5 oz/⅔ cup) granulated sugar
500 ml (17 fl oz/2 cups) apple cider vinegar
Zest and juice of 1 lemon
2 bay leaves
2 teaspoons peppercorns
1 teaspoon salt

METHOD

Collect fresh young seeds from your nasturtium plant, place in the jar and cover with a brine made by mixing the water and salt. Make sure all the seeds are covered. Leave for 24 hours.

Strain off the seeds and dry them gently.

To make the pickling liquid, dissolve the sugar in the vinegar in a saucepan over a low heat. Add the lemon zest and juice, bay leaves, peppercorns and salt, and warm over a low heat for 5 minutes. Allow to cool.

Place the nasturtium seeds in a clean, dry jar. Pour over the cooled pickling liquid.

The pickled seeds will be ready in a couple of weeks and should last 6 months. Keep in the fridge once opened.

Nasturtium & Orange Oxymel

This jewel-coloured sweetened oxymel is bursting with vitamin C and has a very spicy kick. Its expectorant and antibiotic effects make it a must when dealing with colds, sore throats and coughs. Aside from using this oxymel in dressings, you can dilute some in warm water to warm up the whole system.

YOU WILL NEED

Freshly picked nasturtium flowers and leaves (pick on a dry day)
2 strips of orange peel
6 black peppercorns
Apple cider vinegar
Raw honey
Clean, dry, wide-mouthed jar with lid
Natural baking parchment
Labels
Muslin (cheesecloth) and fine-mesh strainer
Storage bottle with lid

METHOD

Fill the jar three-quarters full of nasturtium flowers and leaves and add the orange peel and peppercorns.

Fill the jar to the halfway point with apple cider vinegar. Top with honey. Stir well. Place a square of baking parchment on top of the jar and seal with the lid. Label and leave to infuse for 4–6 weeks.

Strain the oxymel into a jug (pitcher) using a strainer lined with a piece of muslin to remove the flowers. Funnel into a bottle, then label.

The colour of the oxymel will fade over time, but it will last at least 12 months.

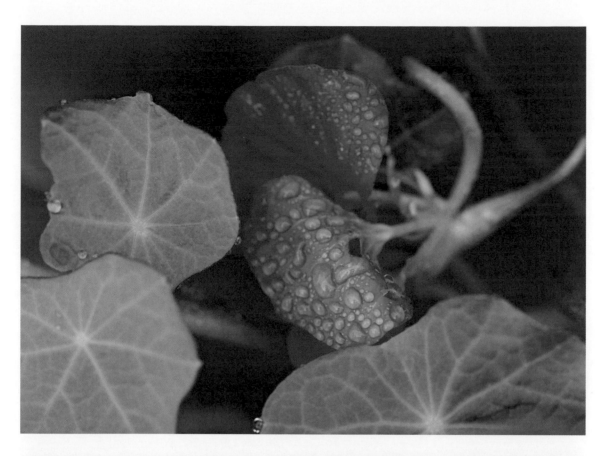

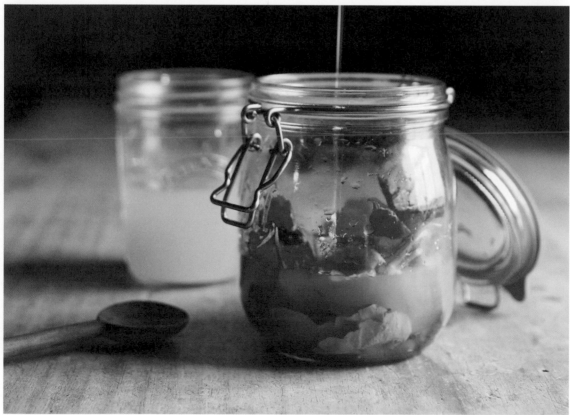

Urtica dioica

Nettle

FAMILY: Urticaceae

PARTS USED: Leaves, seeds and root

ENERGETICS: Cooling and drying

ACTIONS: Alterative, astringent, diuretic, adrenal tonic (seed), anti-allergy, hypotensive, nutritive and tonic

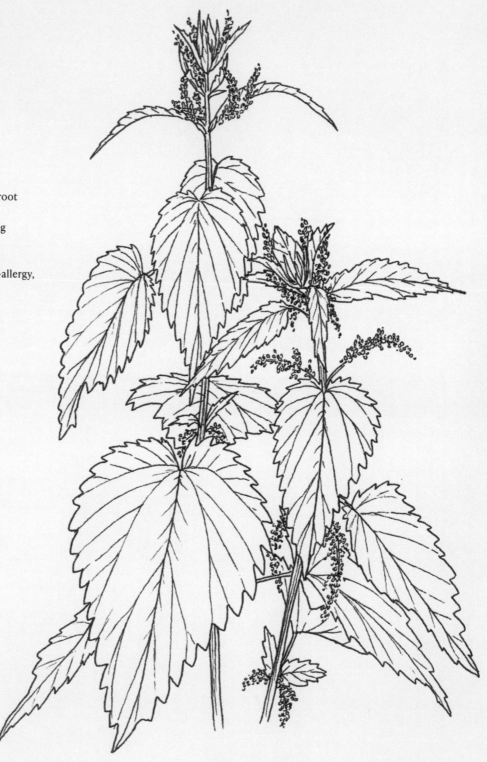

I'm more than slightly infatuated with nettle. It's such a humble-looking plant, dull green with non-distinct flowers and seeds. It would be almost forgettable if it wasn't for its impressive stings. I think it's fair to say nettles are usually plants that many people happily dismiss as unattractive 'weeds' and eagerly remove from the garden, often with the help of weedkillers.

However, once you start discovering the wonders of nettle, you'll never see it as an indistinct weed again. Nettle is actually a very interesting and useful plant that we could all do with befriending, as well as an important plant to support butterflies.

Nettle is readily found on nutrient-rich wasteland. The name derives from the Latin *uro*, meaning 'I burn'. It is said that the nettle came to Britain through the Romans who used this stinging plant to keep themselves warm in the colder climate by using the stings to bring the circulation back into their chilly arms and legs! Traditionally, nettle has been used as a fibre, woven into fabric, as a plant dye and a nutritious food stuff. It can even be made into a hearty, alcoholic brew.

IDENTIFICATION

Nettle is a perennial plant that has heart-shaped leaves with toothed edges. The entire plant is coated in stinging hairs. The flowers are small and indistinct and fall like catkins from the plant, while the seeds hang off the plant in drooping clusters.

USES

Nettles arrive as the perfect tonic herb in spring. It is packed full of minerals and is a wonderful antidote to the lethargy we can feel as we emerge from a long winter season. It contains vitamins A and C, iron, calcium, selenium, zinc, magnesium and potassium, among others, and really is a powerhouse plant. You'll find many tea blends on my kitchen shelves containing this lovely nourishing herb.

Herbalists often use nettle as a general health tonic, especially for women and those who are convalescing, as an adrenal restorer, as an aid against hay fever and allergies, and also for the kidneys and liver.

I love nettle as a mother's tonic – it can help with post-birth bleeding, iron levels and the production of breast milk. It's also gentle and safe to consume during pregnancy as well as after birth.

If you find yourself feeling burnt out and more tired than usual, then nettle is a great restorative remedy. Nettle's tonic-like effect on the body and the seeds' nourishing effects on the adrenals means it's the perfect choice when you're feeling run down and tired by external stresses. A simple tea or infused vinegar are all nice, easy ways to consume nettle daily.

Another great use of nettle is to reduce allergies and, of course, to prevent hay fever. Make a nettle and elderflower infusion and drink daily in the run up to the hay fever season to help lessen the severity of symptoms. Try my Soothing Hay Fever Tea on page 134.

HARVESTING & PREPARATION

Always harvest the young shoots at the top of the plant. Spring is the best time to do this, as older summer nettles aren't great for eating – they can be irritating to our systems and so are best left alone. Make sure you wear gloves while harvesting. If you cut back nettles in spring, you could very well find yourself with a new batch of young growth in summer and certainly in autumn that can be picked again for culinary use, so don't despair if you missed out with the first flush of growth.

You can wilt down nettles and freeze them in batches or dry the leaves for use in teas and tinctures. Nettle should dry well in bunches but, alternatively, you can use a food dehydrator set at approximately 40°C (104°F). Seeds can be collected in summer and pushed through a metal strainer to remove the hairs. They can then be tinctured or eaten as a sprinkle.

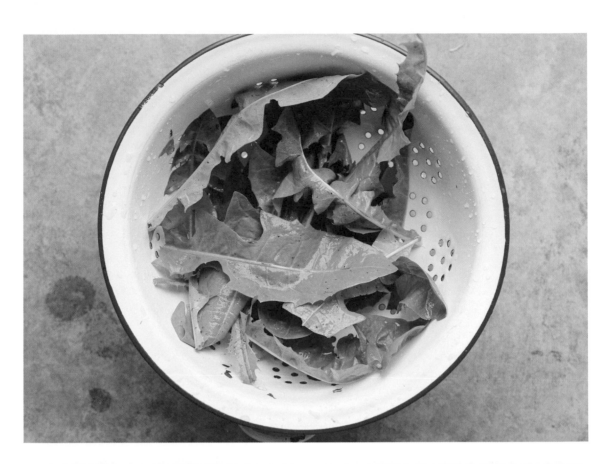

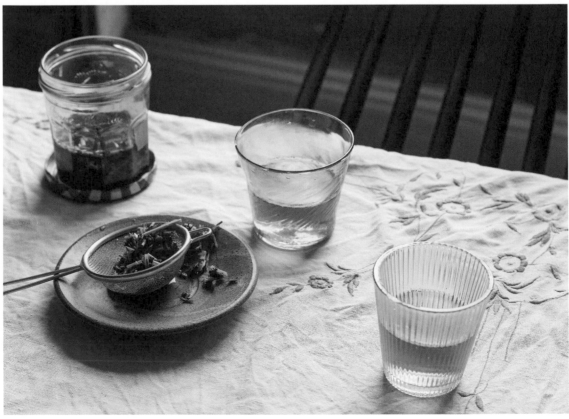

Nettle & Oat Straw Overnight Infusion

This classic combination is one of my favourite teas. The pairing of nettles and oat straw (Avena sativa) is revitalising and nourishing, perfect for helping to support recovery from illness, childbirth or general fatigue.

YOU WILL NEED

1 tablespoon dried nettle leaves
1 tablespoon dried oat straw
Boiling water
Heatproof jar with lid
Fine-mesh strainer

METHOD

Place the nettle and oat straw in the clean, dry jar.

Pour over boiling water, then seal with the lid and allow to infuse overnight before straining into a mug and drinking.

Spring Greens Vinegar

This mineral-rich vinegar is a great addition to salad dressings or taken in warm water as a cleansing tonic. Nettle is the star plant here, but I have also added some dandelion leaves and chickweed for additional benefits. If you don't have access to dandelion and chickweed, just substitute these with extra nettles.

YOU WILL NEED

Freshly picked young nettles, dandelion leaves and chickweed
    (alternatively, dried herbs can be used for a longer shelf life)
Organic apple cider vinegar (containing the mother)
Clean, dry, wide-mouthed jar with lid
Natural baking parchment
Labels
Muslin (cheesecloth) and fine-mesh strainer
Storage bottle with lid

METHOD

Check over the nettles, dandelions and chickweed and ensure they are completely clean.

Chop the plant material. Fill the jar three-quarters full with fresh herbs or half-full if you are using dried herbs, using equal parts of each herb.

Pour over the apple cider vinegar to cover.

Place a square of baking parchment over the mouth of the jar and seal with the lid. Label and allow to infuse for 4 weeks.

Strain the vinegar into a jug (pitcher) using a strainer lined with a piece of muslin to remove the herbal material. Then funnel into the bottle and label.

The vinegar will last up to 6 months if stored in the fridge, but discard at any sign of spoilage.

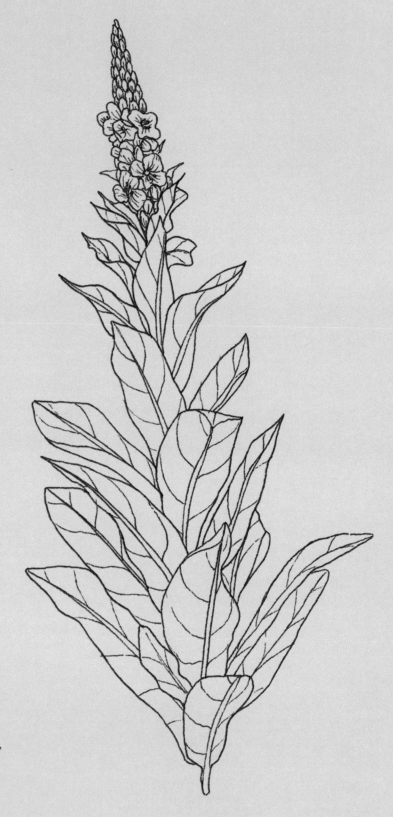

Verbascum thapsus

Mullein

FAMILY: Scrophulariaceae

PARTS USED: Flowers, leaves and roots

ENERGETICS: Cooling

ACTIONS: Anti-inflammatory, antimicrobial, antispasmodic, demulcent, expectorant, vulnerary and anodyne (flowers)

During the initial easing of the lockdown of 2020, I went to visit my parents at their home in County Wicklow, in Ireland. On a walk through their pretty cottage garden, I noticed a huge mullein plant towering over a border close to their house. I enquired why they had planted it in that particular position, to which they replied that they actually hadn't! The mullein had seeded itself right beside their home. Considering mullein is a herb of the lungs, I found this so interesting and very much in keeping with my experience of herbs and their inexplicable ways of being close by when we need them the most.

IDENTIFICATION

The biennial mullein is a visually striking plant. It towers above the rest, reaching up to 2.5 m (8 ft), and has tactile, green-grey leaves coated in soft hairs. The yellow flowers are five-petalled and sit on a long stalk at the top of the plant. They open a few at a time and look a bit like an unripe corn husk to me! Be careful not to confuse mullein with the lethal foxglove.

USES

Mullein, with its soothing and antispasmodic properties, is a wonder herb for lung health. It can calm dry, constant and sore coughs and irritated airways. Due to its anti-inflammatory and demulcent effects, it is often used by herbalists to ease chronic respiratory complaints, including asthma. Traditionally, it was used by doctors as a herbal smoke to open the airways.

Mullein has a gentle expectorant quality that works particularly well for dry coughs where there is inflammation and heat present. The cooling, moistening and anti-inflammatory action of this herb can give relief in these types of coughs. It would also be a nice addition to a hay fever tea.

Personally, I am never without a jar of dried mullein leaves in my home apothecary. I use it mainly in a simple yet powerful tea to ease any respiratory complaints, but make sure you have some coffee filters at hand to remove the not-so-pleasant hairs that come from the leaves.

Mullein also has an affinity with the ears and an infused oil made from the pretty yellow flowers along with fresh garlic is a classic remedy for earache. Mullein flowers have certain anodyne (pain-relieving) qualities that can help with tenderness, while their anti-inflammatory qualities can tackle congestion and general discomfort of the ears. While I personally don't recommend using mullein inside the ear without professional help, I do think massaging around the ear with an infused oil can still be a great way of providing relief.

HARVESTING & PREPARATION

Harvest individual leaves and flowers, but do not strip the plant or it won't survive. Cut the leaves into thick strips and dry on a herb rack or in a food dehydrator set at around 40°C (104°F). Store the dried leaves and flowers in clean, dry, airtight jars out of direct sunlight.

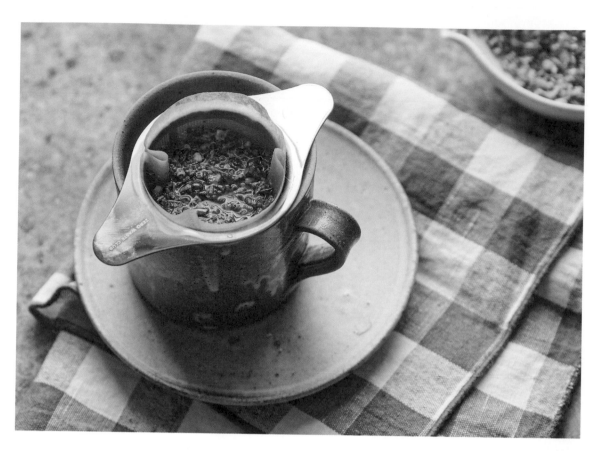

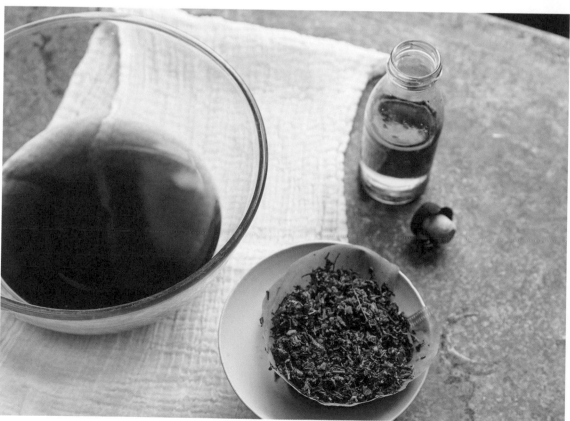

Simple Mullein Tea for Coughs

Mullein tea is something that I reach for when I need powerful respiratory support and as a result I often make this tea during the winter when coughs and colds seem to be rife. It's essential to use a coffee filter when straining the tea as mullein leaves have fine hairs that can be irritating.

YOU WILL NEED

2 teaspoons dried mullein leaves
Boiling water
1 teaspoon raw honey (optional)
Tea strainer and coffee filter

METHOD

Line a tea strainer with a coffee filter and place over a mug. Add the mullein leaves and pour over boiling water.

Allow to steep for 20 minutes, then remove the strainer and filter. It is important to use a fine coffee filter to ensure you remove the irritating hairs, which are very unpleasant to drink – I learnt this the hard way!

Add the honey, stir and drink. Repeat during the day up to three times.

You can also make this infusion using a cold-water overnight infusion. This is an excellent way of making the most of mullein's demulcent qualities.

Mullein & Plantain Cough Syrup

This syrup is perfectly suited for coughs that leave your respiratory system feeling inflamed, dry and unproductive and with a sore throat. Mullein is a gentle expectorant with antimicrobial, anti-inflammatory and antispasmodic properties. Plantain provides soothing relief, while the peppermint cools the heat.

YOU WILL NEED

65 g (2¼ oz/½ cup) dried mullein leaves
32 g (1½ oz/¼ cup) dried plantain leaves
32 g (1½ oz/¼ cup) dried peppermint leaves
500 ml (16 fl oz/2 cups) boiling water
62–125 g (2–4 oz/½–1 cup) raw honey
2 tablespoons brandy
Fine-mesh strainer and coffee filter
Storage bottle with lid
Label

METHOD

Put all the herbs in a heatproof bowl and pour over the boiling water. Leave to infuse for 1–4 hours.

Using a strainer lined with a coffee filter, strain out all the herbs. Remember that mullein has fine hairs, so it's important to use a fine filter for this step.

Measure out 1 cup of herbal liquid. Pour this into a saucepan and add the honey according to taste. Gently warm to combine.

Add the brandy and stir well. Funnel into a bottle and label. Keep refrigerated and use within 4 weeks.

TO USE

Take up to 1 tablespoon when needed during acute situations.

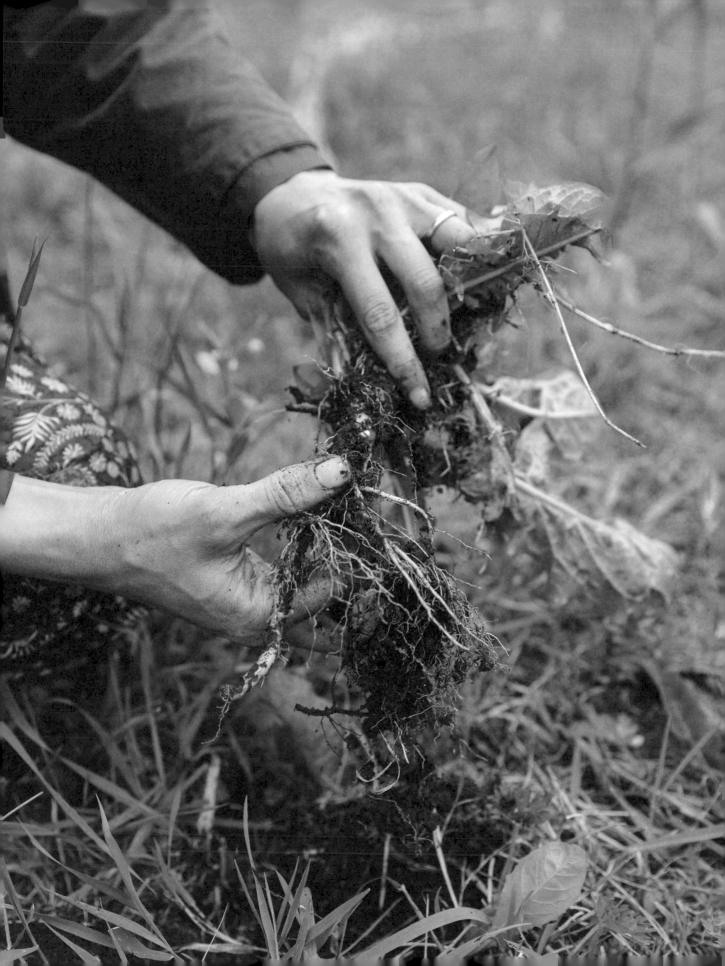

GLOSSARY OF TERMS

Adaptogen: Supportive against stress and its effects on the body.

Alkaloid: A plant constituent that contains nitrogen and is often bitter.

Alterative: Helps to promote balance within the body and cleanses the blood.

Analgesic: Reduces pain.

Anthelmintic: Helps expel worms.

Antibacterial: Reduces or prevents the growth of bacteria

Anti-catarrhal: Helps to shift excess mucous.

Antidepressant: Helps to reduce depression.

Antiemetic: Reduces vomiting and nausea.

Antifungal: Inhibits fungal growth.

Antihistamine: Blocks the histamine response.

Anti-inflammatory: Reduces and soothes inflammation.

Antimicrobial: Inhibits microbial activity.

Antioxidant: Helps to inhibit free radical and oxidative damage.

Antiperspirant: Reduces sweating.

Anti-rheumatic: Relieves discomfort from and helps to prevent rheumatism.

Antiseptic: Halts growth of microbes.

Antispasmodic: Reduces spasms of the muscles.

Antitussive: Helps to stop coughing.

Antiviral: Prevents viruses.

Anxiolytic: Reduces anxiety.

Astringent: Contracts the tissues and mucous membranes.

Bitter: Stimulates digestion through its bitter taste.

Cardiotonic: Tones and strengthens the cardiovascular system.

Carminative: Aids removal of gas and reduces inflammation of the gut.

Cholagogue: Stimulates production of bile.

Decongestant: Reduces mucous.

Demulcent: Soothes irritation and inflammation.

Diaphoretic: Promotes sweating.

Digestive: Aids the digestive system.

Diuretic: Increases urination.

Emmenagogue: Stimulates menstruation.

Emollient: Soothing and protecting.

Energetics: A way of describing the sensorial aspects of a herb.

Expectorant: Supports the respiratory system to expel mucous.

Hepatic: Supports healthy liver function.

Hypotensive: Lowers blood pressure.

Immunomodulator: Strengthens the immune system.

Lymphatic: Helps to encourage healthy movement of lymph.

Mother: The natural cellulose and healthy bacteria included in an unpasteurised vinegar.

Nervine: Lowers anxiety and calms the mind.

Nutritive: Rich in nutrients.

Refrigerant: Has a cooling effect.

Sedative: Relaxing to the nervous system and promotes sleep.

Stimulant: Boosts the activity of the body.

Styptic: Stops external bleeding.

Tonic: Deeply nourishing to the whole body.

Vasodilator: Dilates the blood vessels.

Vulnerary: Healing to the skin.

ABOUT THE AUTHOR

Becky Cole a is forager, home herbalist and gardener living on an ethical, award-winning farm in Northern Ireland. She came across natural living when she was diagnosed with an autoimmune condition and became burnt out with her city life. Since moving to the country, she has become an avid gardener who grows vegetables, herbs and edible flowers and runs popular foraging walks, home apothecary workshops and natural skincare classes. She is the host of the Nature & Nourish podcast and is a regular gardening contributor on BBC Radio 2.

ACKNOWLEDGEMENTS

To the whole team at Hardie Grant who worked alongside me bringing this book to life. It has been a real pleasure to work with such talented, patient and lovely people. Thank you!

To Kim for taking all the photos. It was brilliant fun getting to work together on this and I couldn't have wished for a more talented photographer to team up with.

To Emily for illustrating the herbs with such empathy and delicacy.

To Charlie, Rupert and Toby for being my support and helping to keep me grounded through the whole process from idea to publication.

To Mum and Dad for proofreading the first drafts and always being there for me.

To Cat for being the best sister and friend and keeping me motivated.

To Millie and Robin for letting Charlie and I rewild the land and create Broughgammon on their patch.

To Pam Traill for always encouraging me on my gardening journey, answering questions, bringing me plants and books and allowing us to use her gorgeous garden and woodland at Ballylough.

To Anne and Paddy Casement for allowing us to use their beautiful walled garden. Thank you so much for your generosity!

To my Patreon community for coming along on the journey. You are all amazing! Thank you for your ongoing support.

To Vanessa Feltz and David who gave me an incredible opportunity to share my love of gardening on BBC Radio 2 as a regular contributor. This initially sparked the idea of doing a book in my mind, so thank you!

Finally, to all the gardeners out there doing their bit to grow more plants and befriend the weeds. This book is for you.

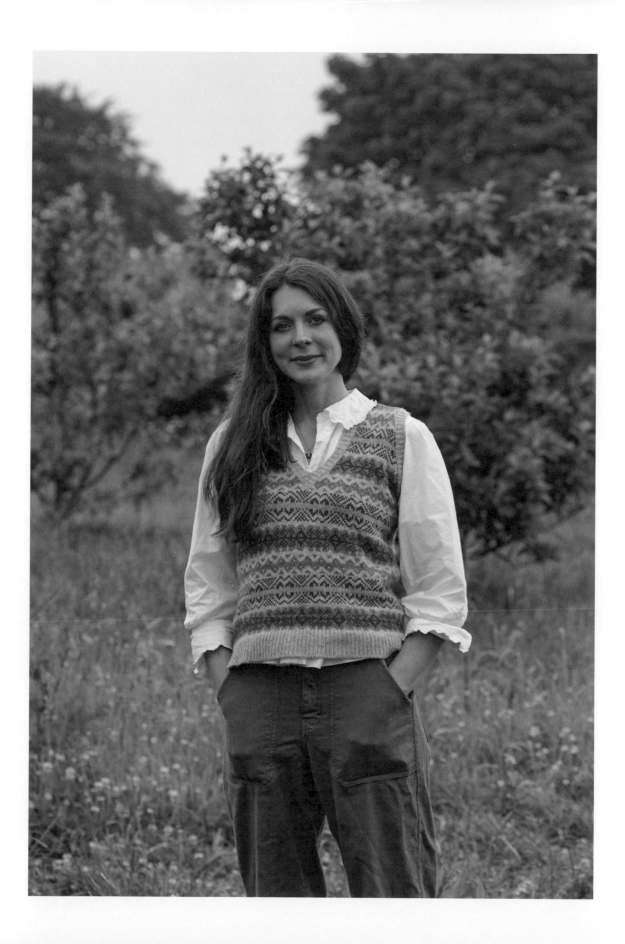

RESOURCES

Herbalist Supplies

UK
G. Baldwin & Co
www.baldwins.co.uk

Jekkas Herbs (for seeds)
www.jekkas.com

USA
Mountain Rose Herbs
www.mountainroseherbs.com

Further Reading

Anne McIntyre, *The Complete Herbal Tutor*, Aeon Books, 2019

David Hoffman, *Medical Herbalism: The Science and Practice of Herbal Medicine*, Healing Arts Press, 2003

James Green, *The Herbal Medicine-Maker's Handbook*, Crossing Press, 2000

Kim Walker and Vicky Chown, *The Handmade Apothecary*, Kyle Books, 2017

Maria Groves, *Body into Balance: An Herbal Guide to Holistic Self-Care*, Storey Publishing, 2016

Marlow Renton and Eric Briggane, *Foraging Pocket Guide*, Otherwise, 2019

Richard Maybe, *Food for Free*, Collins, 2012

Robert Tisserand and Rodney Young, *Essential Oil Safety*, Elsevier, 2013

Robin Rose Bennett, *The Gift of Healing Herbs*, North Atlantic Books, 2014

Robin Wall, *Braiding Sweetgrass*, Penguin, 2020

Rosemary Gladstar, *Medicinal Herbs: A Beginner's Guide*, Storey Publishing, 2012

Rosallee de la Forêt, *Alchemy of Herbs*, Hay House, 2017

Thomas J. Elpel, *Botany in a Day: The Patterns Method of Plant Identification*, HOPS Press, 2013

Keep in Touch

www.beckyocole.com My website with details of my online courses and in-person workshops.